Contents

Foreword

We have all had teachers who have been important to us. In my case it was Mr DeJarnett, my high school algebra teacher. Math appears to be exact, unambiguous: there is a single right answer; there are correct ways to proceed; there is no room for creativity. But Mr DeJarnett somehow helped us discover the magic in numbers. He encouraged us to invent what he called 'short-cuts'. He made us feel like pioneers in the field. We often left class celebrating our conquest of a particularly stubborn equation. When I look back, I realize that he was a coach.

I can't help but believe that he was having fun in the classroom, I know his students were. We talked about algebra at lunchtime and after school. Many of us even entered universities as math majors, only to abandon the field when we found that Mr DeJarnett was a bit of an anomaly in the world of mathematics. But even though we did not pursue careers in math, Mr DeJarnett did significantly impact our lives. Without knowing it, he introduced me to my profession, he taught me to coach.

Back in the 1960s when I was in my algebra class, there was not a specific term for what this teacher was doing. He was just teaching, albeit in an unconventional way. But his consistent results attracted the attention of teachers and administrators. Test scores were higher than expected and, perhaps more importantly, students were excited — about algebra of all things!

I wonder what Mr DeJarnett would say about (what was natural for him) this thing called coaching which has now become a recognized profession. For him coaching was simply a way to interest us in algebra. Today coaching has become a method that encourages us to seek, to explore our potential, to awaken that which has been present but hidden within us.

This book reveals precisely what Mr DeJarnett was doing, and what many exceptional teachers intuitively do. It provides practical ways to bring coaching into the classroom. At its core, coaching is about curiosity. It is about pondering and searching and trying and failing and having that failure feed our curiosity so that we try again.

An effective coach cultivates an atmosphere of exploration and discovery. Every explorer unavoidably takes wrong turns. A good quest invariably includes difficulties. Coaching not only recognizes the inevitability of failure, but celebrates that failure for the growth that comes in its wake. In the space of coaching, there is not room for judgment or self-recrimination. Mistakes are part of the journey, giving us more information and moving us along, even when they appear to take us down an unproductive path.

Just imagine how many hands would go up in the classroom if none of the students worried about 'getting it wrong' or looking foolish. Throughout life, how often do *we* fail to 'put our hands up'? How often as adults are we stuck in inaction because of fear or self-doubt?

Coaching is about learning throughout life in a natural and positive way. As human beings, we want to learn. We love to explore. We have an innate desire to grow and develop. We are curious. Coaching engages that curiosity. That is what the Mr DeJarnetts of the world really do. They encourage us to eagerly put our hands up.

Jan Elfline EdD MCC
Jan Elfline Limited
Bloomington, IL, USA
www.janelfline.com
July 2005

Foreword

In the cloistered world inhabited by educational theorists, it is something of a truism to assert that 'assessment drives learning'. In other words, students learn what will get them through their exams. Or, to be more precise, they learn what they *think* will get them through their exams. Those with their hands on the rudder of medical education use this phenomenon quite deliberately. As a former Convenor of the MRCGP examination I know how, by instituting a Critical Reading Question in the 1990s, we sensitised a generation of GP registrars to the principles of evidence-based medicine while, at the same time, by including some questions on classic books about general practice in the written paper, we signalled that a GP's understanding of human experience should draw upon a broader evidence base than is reported in the *BMJ* and the *BJGP*.

Truth is usually more complicated than truisms, however. It would be truer to say that every form of assessment fosters *some* kinds of learning but discourages others. Assess young doctors' communication skills with a written test, for example, and what they learn is to quote the standard references and to trot out somebody else's summary of the usual models. Use video recordings or simulated patients for the same purpose, and there is a danger that what sets out to be a test of patient-centred consulting may, in weaker students, encourage not empathy but play-acting. The phenomenon of 'perverse incentives', an unfortunate consequence of a target-driven NHS, is equally rife in medical education.

General practice is currently in the grip of a soul-wrenching paradox. Its science base has never been stronger; yet, to patients adrift in an impersonal sea of information, its human touch has never been more precious. There is a simultaneous clamour for regulation and accountability on one hand, and respect for individual choice and autonomy on the other. Our professional performance, it seems, must be standardised, audited, outcome-based. At the same time it must be subtle and flexible, taking account of all the unpredictabilities of the human condition. We know we should be un-compromising in pursuit of that homogenised version of 'best practice' set out in a mountain of protocols and guidelines so high that it blots out the sun. Yet everything in us protests that general practice is nothing if it is not rooted in concern for the uniqueness of that other person who brings for our attention a singular story, a singular predicament.

The trick we have to bring off is not to see rigour and individuality as opposites. Predictability and unpredictability can coexist. It is possible for science to wear a human face, and for compassion to be deployed in a rational way. As the RCGP motto puts it, '*Cum scientia caritas*'. Good GPs achieve this synthesis a dozen times every surgery. It's not hard; the trick is knowing that it matters.

It matters just as much in education. Another truism: the relationship between teacher and pupil mirrors that between doctor and patient in its fundamental dynamics. In both, it is the quality of attention paid by the helper to the helped that is crucial. The same paradox is there in the educational domain as in the clinical. Much of what passes for professional development is either over-structured 'teaching to curriculum' or sloppy 'learning by whim'. And the trick we have to bring off is to blend rigour with insight, learner-centredness with objectivity.

It can be done. Just as patients are best helped by well-informed doctors who can nevertheless put their own agendas second, so learners best flourish and grow if their teachers can overcome a 'teacher knows best' didacticism, and instead offer a light – 'I'm curious as to why you think ...' or 'What would happen if you tried ... ?'

Are there such teachers? Yes of course; they're called coaches. Sports coaches are nothing new; 'life coaches' are still sufficiently novel to be amusing. But the 'coaching' model of education – teaching by asking the right questions – has been with us since the time of Socrates. And coaching works. To be coached by someone who knows what they're doing is a liberating and invigorating experience. Ask any Wimbledon champion. Can coaching be taught? Probably. I guess you have to start from a genuine desire to be effective, and to put your effectiveness genuinely at the disposal of the learner. That said, there are methods and techniques, principles and procedures, which can make the would-be coach as effective as possible. This book is a *vade mecum* of systematic coaching practice, and will bring the necessary intellectual discipline to the good intentions the reader may be assumed to possess.

One final truism: 'the medium is the message'. Coaching, if widely adopted as the prevailing model of continuing professional development, would result in us doctors taking much better care of each other – not in an introverted 'you scratch *my* back ...' way, but as a way of keeping our professional skills and values in the best possible condition to help our patients. Three messages resound throughout this text. Firstly, curiosity is a good thing for coaches (and doctors) to cultivate. Secondly, learners (and patients) are intrinsically self-directing and self-motivating. Thirdly, although there may be a formal relationship between coach and pupil (or doctor and patient), the best things happen if the parties are free not to behave in formulaic or role-determined ways.

These messages are not truisms. I think they are the truth.

Roger Neighbour MA DSc FRCP PRCGP
President, Royal College of General Practitioners
Author of *The Inner Consultation* and *The Inner Apprentice*[1,2]
Bedmond, Hertfordshire
July 2005

References

1 Neighbour R (2004) *The Inner Consultation: how to develop an effective and intuitive coaching style* (2e). Radcliffe Publishing, Oxford.

2 Neighbour R (2004) *The Inner Apprentice: an awareness-centred approach to vocational training for general practice* (2e). Radcliffe Publishing, Oxford.

Preface

Why have we chosen to write a book about coaching and how its methods can be used to help others learn? Fundamentally, it is because we are passionate about the value of coaching in developing the skills of lifelong learning. We have used these techniques and we have witnessed the impact they have on the learner, the teacher and their relationship. We have felt for some time that as teaching and learning become more focused on assessment and structure, some of the essence of learning has been lost. It is right that a learner should ensure that they know what they have to know, and that those who will benefit from their learning, their future clients, can be assured that the person who will be working with them is appropriately skilled, and knows what they are talking about. We feel, however, that this tends to distract from some of the really valuable parts of the learning process – of the learner discovering about themselves; what makes them tick; how they learn best; why they get into the same pickle over and over again; how they repeat ways of doing things that have worked in the past, and transfer those strategies into other parts of their life; how they can self-motivate, and remain enthusiastic. These are the skills that are crucial to continuing professional and personal development. These are the skills that will maintain professional standards and wisdom in the face of overwhelming information growth.

As learning has become more systematised and task driven, it has a tendency to become separate from other parts of a learner's life. We wanted to suggest ways that would help trainers get the best of both worlds, help learners develop as people and as thinkers, as well as helping them be the best at their job they could possibly be.

Using strategies that come out of coaching can really help. We know that many of us already use in our teaching much of what we have written about, but at an unconscious level. As discussed in the chapter on modelling (Chapter 9), moving strategies from the unconscious to the conscious means that they are accessible to us whenever we choose to use them. And having more choice in how we teach will, we believe, make us better teachers. As Abraham Maslow is reputed to have said, if the only tool you have is a hammer, you treat everything like a nail. We hope you discover an ironmongery of tools!

Maria-Teresa Claridge
Tony Lewis
July 2005

About the authors

Dr Maria-Teresa Claridge is a family doctor and general practitioner (GP) trainer in a small rural practice on Dartmoor in Devon. She has been actively involved in education for over 10 years with experience in developing and delivering postgraduate courses, running small groups and teaching and coaching on a one-to-one basis. Her passion has always been the psychology of health and communication skills. This passion combined with a sense that there was more than traditional educational models offered, and that she wanted to broaden her own skills to help her adopted children led her to study neurolinguistic programming (NLP). She is a master NLP practitioner and accredited NLP coach. She uses her NLP coaching skills in all areas of her life. The motivation for writing the book comes from a belief that in the face of an overwhelming information boom there should be a balancing emphasis to develop and enhance the process of teaching.
Email: mt.heather@tesco.net; marie-theresa.claridge@gp-L83082.nhs.uk

Dr Tony Lewis is a family doctor in Exmouth, Devon for some of the week. The rest of the time he works as a teaching fellow in the Peninsula Medical School and also as associate director in general practice postgraduate training in the South West Peninsula Deanery. He has always been interested in helping others learn, and was appointed a trainer in general practice in the seventies, following this by being a GP course organiser in Cornwall for seven years, and then regional adviser in general practice for Devon and Cornwall. For 10 years he also directed the MSc in healthcare at Exeter University. This has given Tony a wide experience of one-to-one teaching, as well as small group facilitation and lecturing to larger audiences. A fascination in discovering how others do what they do led him to becoming a master practitioner in NLP, and then an accredited NLP coach. Tony feels that developing learning through coaching has not only enhanced the work he does as a small group facilitator and one-to-one teacher, it has also changed the way he works as a doctor, and affected other areas of his life.
Email: tony@tonyplewis.com

Acknowledgements

We would like to thank Ian McDermott and Jan Elfline for their inspirational teaching. We are particularly grateful to Jan for her support and encouragement as we have integrated and developed coaching with GP trainers in the southwest. As always we have learned most from the doing and the teaching and we would like to thank all who have learnt, and will continue to learn, with us.

1

Introduction

So what is coaching?

Coaching is a word used in many different arenas and so you may come to this book with many preconceptions about what coaching is. Sports coaches help people do amazing things at the Olympics. Students who do not do too well at school may be coached to improve their performance. The concept of personal and professional coaching is gathering ground in many areas of business and teaching. Coaching is also sometimes seen as a form of therapy or counselling. Coaching and mentoring too, are often confused, though the overlap here is much more marked and both can use similar strategies. So what are the similarities and differences between all these things? Coaching and mentoring are probably the two most similar forms of support for development, and often use the same processes. Mentoring typically involves a colleague in the same line of business who can act as a guide, sponsor or support for a less experienced person, whereas a coach need not necessarily be in the same line of business as the person they are coaching. Coaching, we feel, is definitely not therapy or counselling. This is a trap that therapists who become teachers can sometimes fall into, and adopting a coaching style of working could encourage. As we discuss in the chapter on 'designing the alliance' (Chapter 3), it is a good idea to actually write into the contract that you will not be counselling. Boundaries are important in coaching, and there is a clear boundary between coaching and therapy.

For us coaching in the learning context is about enabling a learner to develop in the best way for them at the time, and to enable them to evaluate the choices open to them in order to move forward. It is about getting the 'learning how to learn' internalised so that it becomes part of the person for life.

And what happens in coaching?

Coaching is about working with people to help them be more effective in what they want to do. It works with a person's own agenda rather than that of the coach. A coach rarely gives advice, rather works with a person by challenging, probing and asking questions.

There are several presuppositions about coaching. The first is the coach presumes that the learners themselves are resourceful; they have the means and understanding to help themselves solve their own problems. The essence here is that only the individuals themselves know the full story. It is they who have to put into operation any agreed actions. They know what they can and cannot do. The coach acts by helping people find those inner resources and by helping them realise that they can use them effectively, often by helping them work with limiting beliefs.

The second is that the learner sets their own agenda. This means that the agenda is intensely focused around areas which are important to the learner, and only the learner themself can know what those areas are. This relates closely to ideas developed from the concepts of adult learning espoused by Knowles and others.[1] The challenge for a trainer is to know that there is a professional agenda as well, and to steer a path between meeting that agenda and working with the learner's agenda.

The third is to know that you, the trainer as coach, and your learner are equals. This is discussed in more detail in the chapter on building the alliance between you as coach and your coachee (Chapter 3). This relationship of equals is fundamental. As one of the premises is that your coachee has all the resources within themself to solve their issues, it is axiomatic that they are as resourceful as you in dealing with their own problems, which means that the relationship between the two of you must be equal.

The fourth is to realise that your learner comes with a history, a past, as well as a future. Good coaches realise that issues learners bring up in the present are affected by what happened to them in the past, as well as by what their aspirations and goals are in the future. To work fully with your learner requires you to take notice of these things and treat the person as a whole.

Finally, coaching is about action, it is about helping your learner do something. This requires commitment from both parties. It requires commitment from you to work within the broad framework of coaching, and requires commitment from the learner to explore places where they need to change. Both of these can sometimes be quite uncomfortable. Change is always challenging, but change when you have a coach at your side is exciting.

So what is different about this approach to learning? Training, teaching and coaching all appear to be about learning. The main difference is that in the coaching environment the learner themself does the exploring. They find out what they need to know. They find resources both externally and internally. Sometimes you as the coach may turn out to be the resource they are looking for. But the learner will have decided what it is they need from you, and how they will use the material. This can at times be quite stressful for you as coach — you know what they should do to change things. You know what they need to know that will make all the difference. And you may well be right. Often though, by not knowing the full picture, or by not knowing the complete context of that learning for the learner, you will get it wrong.

Exercise

Think of a good learning experience you had some time in the past.

Really get into that experience, live it for real, and as you do that, see what you see, hear what you hear and feel what you feel.

What was the experience like? How was it good? What were the features of it that really worked for you?

Now think of a learning experience that was not good.

Again really get into that experience — or, if that is too uncomfortable, see it as if it were happening to someone else, as if you are standing back from it.

Again, what was the experience like? How was it not so good? What were the features of it that really jarred for you?

The guess is that the good experience had features where you were in charge, you felt valued, you knew what you wanted, and you were energised by the process and came away from it feeling you could do anything. And the bad experience was something about feeling small, feeling incompetent and useless, about feeling you would never get a handle on how to do it right, about never seeing yourself as being OK.

We believe that adopting a coaching frame of mind and of being, when you are teaching and helping others learn is more likely to produce good learning experiences. Try the strategies we offer in this book, and see what happens. As is said in neurolinguistic programming, try them on for size and see if they fit. We think you can walk a mile in these shoes, and what a fantastic mile it will be ...

How to get the most from this book

This book will be of value to you whether you are teaching on a one-to-one apprenticeship model or in small groups. Many of the chapters will also be useful to those of you who lecture to hundreds of students at a time. As teacher to yourself and to your children, this book will also be a valuable tool.

You will know how you get the most from books; you may flick through to get a flavour and then read sequentially; or you may be a 'dipper in and out' – or you may read cover to cover. We have written this book as a 'how to' manual, it is practical rather than theoretical. We suggest that you approach this book with an open and curious mind, and that as you read you stop and think about real cases, teaching scenarios that you personally have been involved in. The exercises that we have used are essential to the learning process – they will enable you to shift from conscious competence to unconscious competence. Take the time to do them and to answer the questions honestly for yourself, knowing that there are no right or wrong answers. Remember also that you are a learner too, be open to the learning as you teach and notice what challenges you; where you flow easily; where you are surprised; where you have fun and where you do not. Keep a note of these times and come back to the book and the exercises to discover what the stretch is for you. Above all, remember that you are human – this may all sound obvious, but the doing is harder than the reading. Practise one new thing at a time and allow yourself to have fun and enjoy the learning.

Reference

1   Knowles M (1984) *The Adult Learner: A Neglected Species* (3e). Gulf Publishing, Houston, TX.

2

Curiosity-coaching for learning: a different state to learn from

Remember as a child the excitement of special treats, the anticipation of receiving a gift. The curiosity of wanting to know now, hunting in your parents' favourite hiding place for that present, prying open the wrapping of parcels then trying to stick it all back together before you were found out. That's curiosity.

Curiosity suggests playfulness, it is open and inviting. It is non-judgemental. Consider a baby learning to walk or exploring its environment, where despite the bumps it keeps on going and trying again. As adults learning a new skill we give up more easily, informed as we are by an educational culture of right and wrong. The art of curious wondering and trying different ways is often much harder for the adult. How often have you heard the learner paralysed in fear of judgement ask 'yes, but what is the right way?'.

Suspend judgement and wonder instead

We use judgement every day of our lives, we have to in order to decide what to pursue or what to avoid. However, there is a potential danger in the rapid and rigid judgements that are so often required of any professional. We tend to use stereotypes and we put up 'either/or' choices to justify our own or others' positions. The danger of judgement in learning and development is two-fold, in the rejection and in the acceptance. Something rejected vanishes from our perception and attention; it is difficult for it to resurface in our thinking. Equally, something may be accepted so unquestioningly that there is no room for options and flexibility related to person or circumstance.

We are well aware of the dilemmas this creates in real life where there are rarely completely right or completely wrong answers. For many learners, particularly those trained in deductive or scientific methods, the measure of achievement is in the ability to be 'right'. For these learners, the loss of curiosity and creativity about themselves and the world is the price they have paid. With increasing experience, professionals acknowledge the importance of wisdom in decision making, of being open to wider meaning, and trusting intuition. To trust intuition, which comes from the unconscious learning that comes through experience, and to practise wisdom, requires an open mind. Coaching gives permission to suspend judgement and to put the curiosity back into professional and personal learning.

Wondering

Curiosity starts with a question: 'I wonder what …?'; 'I wonder if …?'; 'I wonder how …?'.

It invites us to go looking. It is wondering and exploring. It invites options. It is not information gathering or point scoring. Curious questions are open questions, and questions that invite deeper thought. They are best prefaced conversationally by 'I'm curious' or 'I'm interested'.

Let us consider the following example of discussing a project with a learner. There are two forms of questions we may ask – one is open and curious, the other is more limiting in possible responses. A good analogy is that a curious question is like setting off down a series of branching tunnels; at each point you make a choice and then move forward to the next junction. A purely information-seeking question ends in a blind alley, no way to go forward. A curious question presupposes an unconditional sense that the answer is the right one for the learner at that time. It enables an answer to be challenged and opens the door to further questions.

Both forms of question have value. As you compare the questions consider the nature of the responses you may get. Who is making the decision? Who is learning and moving forward effectively . . . the learner or the coach? What is the value for ongoing learning? For many teachers, their natural tendency is to ask information-seeking questions. By increasing our repertoire of questions we increase our flexibility and our usefulness to our learners. Table 2.1 gives examples of questions to ask about doing a project.

As a coach demonstrating curiosity by questioning and suspending judgement, you do not presuppose solutions or right and wrong answers. As a coach, you invite a journey and you provide leverage for change. This is the cornerstone of effective professional and personal learning.

Table 2.1   Questions to ask about doing a project

Data gathering	Curious
What ideas have you for a project?	What do you want out of this project? How do you want to feel at the end of the project? What is the best project for you to do now?
Which of the two options will you choose?	What is another choice you could make in addition?
Is this a good way of doing it?	What makes this a good way of doing it for you?
How much time do you need?	What do you need in order to do this? How are you going to ensure you do this as well as you can? What is the first step?
Why aren't you getting on with it?	What's stopping you? What do you need in order to move forward? What is this all about? What do you need to say no to?

Tolerating confusion and uncertainty

Some of us tolerate uncertainty better than others. We devise different mechanisms for dealing with confusion and uncertainty in our lives. Almost by definition, the state of learning is one of confusion and uncertainty. Curiosity tolerates confusion and uncertainty, and welcomes it as the path to understanding.

Exercise

How are you with confusion and uncertainty?

This is a good exercise as a coach and as a learner.

Think of a time when you feel confused or uncertain. It may be arriving in an unknown country and having to arrange transport or accommodation, maybe completing a tax form or reading a legal document. It may be facing a new professional contract over which you have no control or it may be in a relationship where you sense things are not going well but you don't know why or what to do next.

Notice how you react to the confusion and uncertainty. Make notes:

- Do you feel negative and want to push it away?

or

- Do you enjoy wondering how you will fit all the pieces together and what you will do next?

Ask yourself:

- What happens when I'm not in control?
- How well do I tolerate uncertainty?
- How do I feel when I'm confused?
- What images, sounds or self-talk comes to mind when I am confused?

- How do you know when you are not confused?
- How do you know when you are certain?

To be confused or uncertain you have to have some information, a partial understanding. If you are totally ignorant or simply don't know something, you cannot be confused. So confusion viewed with a curious mind is a great opportunity for learning. A coach will acknowledge the confusion and then challenge what it is all about in order to move forward. Here it is useful to look at an example of working with a learner who is confused.

Example

Handling confusion

Coachee: I am so muddled I really don't know what to do
Coach: That's OK, it's OK to be confused. Let's unpick the confusion and see how you can move forward.
Coachee: Unpick confusion, um ...
Coach: There are many areas to be confused about ... for example you may be confused because:

- there is missing *information*
- you don't know *what* to do
- you don't know *how* to do something
- it conflicts with your *beliefs* and values
- it is not in keeping with your *sense of self*.

Coachee: Well I don't actually know what the guidelines say about this, and also I'm not sure I can actually break that sort of news.

> *Coach*: So having more information will help?
> *Coachee*: Yes.
> *Coach*: And what's this about 'can' you break this news. I'm interested —
> is that about the 'how to' or is that about what you think is the right
> thing to do?
> *Coachee*: No, it's OK for me to do it — that's my job; it's about how to
> do it well.
> *Coach*: OK, now we've got something to work with. What is the first
> step? What would help you now?

Next time you are confused ask yourself 'in which of the five areas am I confused?', and notice how you feel different. Try them with a learner, notice how things move forward constructively, and notice who is in the driving seat.

The importance of curiosity in the relationship

By incorporating the model of coaching into your teaching you are giving very important messages to your learner. The curious coach does not have all the answers, but rather comes as a collaborator in the search for options and possibilities. The assumption is that the learner has the resources to come up with the best solution for themselves at the time. Learning that is cultivated in this climate is most likely to be sustained and developed.

Authentic curiosity allows the learner to reveal themselves in a safe non-threatening environment. Imagine meeting a new person at a party who is really curious about who you are, what makes you tick, your interests and values. Not only are you likely to be flattered, but you may also find yourself questioning and making new connections about your life. The same questions asked in an interrogative way by someone who shows no interest in the answers will have a very different effect; most likely you will put up your defences, to them and yourself.

If you are in a really curious state you will be genuinely interested in how it is for the learner. You will have an open frame where you do not anticipate or assume the responses your learner will give. You will find yourself being truly interested and asking yourself:

- How did they do that?
- What was going through their head as they did that?

- I wonder what would convince them?
- What is this all about for them?

The focus of your listening will not be what this all means for you and how you did something similar to what they did. Rather your listening will be truly active, focused on the learner's words, the meaning behind them, their body language, emotion, pace and energy. To be truly listened to is a very honouring experience. It is what we aspire to in all our relationships.

The power of curiosity in a learning relationship is that it is highly contagious. The learner starts to develop the skills for themselves. Questions become more powerful and more intriguing. The learner learns what it's like to be curious about themselves, to be less judgemental and more tolerant. And that is a great recipe for personal and professional development.

So how do you get into a curious state?

A state is your way of being at a particular moment. States change continuously, and we are often not consciously aware of what state we are in. State is manifest by the way we talk and behave – our physical and emotional energy. We may even say in common parlance, 'There's no need to get in such a state!'

You know how a particular state has a specific set of triggers – for example a smell, a tone of voice or a photograph can trigger warm happy feelings, and you can find yourself smiling involuntarily. Know also that you can self-trigger and set a state at will. The most familiar example of this is taking deep breaths, hearing your favourite piece of music or visualising a tranquil scene in order to calm down and generate a relaxed state.

As a coach it is very beneficial to work with a frame of curiosity and to develop this state. You may already be a curious and interested person when you are in a teaching or training situation. If so, consider the following exercise as a way of developing the skill still further. If curiosity is not a natural teaching/training state this is a start.

Exercise

1 *Set your intention to be curious.* Say to yourself I am going to be curious, really interested in what makes this person tick. I am going to suspend judgement for the next few minutes.

2 *Spend fifteen minutes sitting quietly observing someone.* Maybe in a work situation, teaching or in a café or shop. Don't talk – just watch and

yourself: 'I wonder what they believe?', 'I wonder what they enjoy about work?', 'What gives them satisfaction?', 'What motivates them?', 'What does that behaviour say about their values?'

3 *Now be curious about you.* How did that feel? Was it easy? Was it difficult? What made it so? How could you be more curious? And if you were more curious what would that give you?

4 *Set your own anchor or trigger.* What will remind you of this state: a colour, a picture, a memory of a time when you were absorbed in fascination, a sound, a way of sitting or holding your hands, or it may be reminding yourself to set the intention.

5 *Recreate this state and see yourself in this state in the future with your learner.*

Practise this as many times as possible.

Now that you can create a curious state, start practising asking some curious questions in this state. Remember they are not data-seeking questions, but questions that lead one to another that encourage rambling and depth.

Remember to preface your questions with: 'I am interested ...'; 'I am curious ...'; 'I wonder ...'

Notice what happens. If there are silences, pauses and reflections, you know that you are asking powerful curious questions (see Chapter 6, on tools and techniques). If you sense yourself opening and letting go of judgement you are working in a curious state.

Curiosity about learning

Coaching encourages and develops significant, meaningful, experiential learning. Carl Rogers asserted that experiential learning has five qualities: it involves thought and feelings; it is self-initiated, with a sense of discovery coming from within; it is pervasive and makes a difference in the behaviour, attitudes and possibly the personality of the learner; the learner knows if their needs have been met or not; and finally it has meaning.[1] The teacher, or coach in our terms, is primarily concerned with encouraging and allowing the learner to learn from their own curiosity. The result is the wisdom and skill to apply knowledge appropriately. This is particularly pertinent in many areas with the current explosion in knowledge.

In order to fulfil the maximum potential for personal and professional learning certain criteria have to be met. Maslow's hierarchy of needs describes how in order to move to this level, lower level needs such as security and comfort must first be partially satisfied.[2] Csikszentimihalyi described the sensation of optimal experience or flow where there is a balance between the challenges perceived in a given situation and the skills a person brings to it.[3] It is an experience often described as the 'merging of activity and awareness', in which there is a lack of self-awareness, time becomes distorted and there is a transcendence of self. 'Flow' is intrinsically rewarding. It is an enjoyable experience that people seek to replicate, and that improves learning and performance

So how can we tap into all this and how can we help the learner learn in the most effective way for them? There are many models and tools used in education. For example Honey and Mumford's learning styles show us our preferred style between activist, theorist, pragmatist and reflector.[4] Other models refer to a preference in senses, for example visual, auditory or kinaesthetic. These models give an insight and a useful handle into an aspect of learning. However they do not reflect the beauty of the whole. It is like describing a sunset as orange and pink.

For the coach, the prime interest is not in fitting the learner into a box, leaning back and saying, 'Well, there you go, all visual pragmatists do that. What can you expect?' Rather the coach is curious about what learning actually means for the individual. They wonder, 'How does this person learn most effectively? What do they need more of? What do they need less of?' The coach opens the door for the learner to acknowledge and recognise aspects of their own learning which they may not have previously been conscious of.

So in addition to the various educational and psychological tools, here are some examples of questions you may ask:

- What do you think/believe about learning?
- What do you think/believe about your ability to learn?
- What do you think/believe about feedback?

- Think of a time when you learnt well … what made it good?
- How do you learn best? What do you see, hear and feel?
- What do you need to learn the best you can?

- Think of a time when learning wasn't so good … what was that all about?
- What inhibits your learning?
- So when you notice that happening what will you do?

- What motivates you to learn?
- What demotivates you?
- What do you find easy to remember?
- How do you remember?

- What do you tend to forget?
- What does that tell you?

- How do you want to learn?
- What is the first step?
- When will you do that?
- What can you do today that will help?
- Will you?

You can practise asking these questions of anyone – friends, family your children. Notice how they may need to 'go inside' for the answers, notice their interest and yours. There is no need to pass comment – just accept the answer as it comes.

And finally, the 'yes but' . . . curiosity without answers

It is often said that 'curiosity killed the cat' and a common reaction to the sorts of questions we have been using here is 'Help! What if I don't know the answer?' or 'What if I know the answer, it's obvious what they should do?' In transactional analysis terms these concerns suggest a frame where the coach is OK, but the learner is not OK and needs mending or fixing. The coach/learner relationship is not about this; learner and coach are both OK; they are both expert and resourceful. This state of curiosity and non-judgement is a most powerful tool to maintain this equality. It enables the learner to tap into their own resources and find their own connections and solutions. And these connections and solutions are the 'right' ones for that person at that time. Curiosity without answers gives us freedom, tolerance and respect in our learning.

References

1   Rogers C and Freiburg HJ (1993) *Freedom to Learn* (3e) Merrill, New York.

2   Maslow A (1968) *Toward a Psychology of Being*. D Van Nostrand Company, New York.

3   Csikszentimihalyi M (1966) *Creativity: flow and the psychology of discovery and invention*. Harper Collins, New York.

4   Honey P and Mumford A. Learning styles questionnaire www.peterhoney.com (accessed 20 May 2005).

3

Building the relationship between coach and learner: designing the alliance

Traditionally, teaching and training was about telling students what they needed to know. As the teacher, we knew what the curriculum was; we had our own agenda. The power here was with the teacher. As the concept of adult learning gained ground, teachers worked with the students' agenda, discovered their learning outcomes, and empowered them to find the resources in themselves to answer the questions. Power moved to the student. In the coaching relationship, power rests neither with the coach, nor really with the coachee, but in the relationship between the two.

So the relationship you have with your learner is fundamental to the success of teaching. A good relationship will increase the learning your client gets, as well as making it much more enjoyable for you as the teacher. Designing the alliance you have with your learner is part of making this successful. It is an alliance, in that both you as teacher and the other as learner are deeply involved in making it work, and between you both, you mould the alliance to meet the needs of the learner.

This means that the success of your coaching depends very much on the relationship that you have with your learner, which in turn means that your learner determines the success of the coaching. This also means that one of your vital functions as coach is to work on how the relationship you have with your coachee can serve you both. Shifting this attention away from you as a teacher can be uncomfortable at first. It may be a new way for you to experience teaching. It may entail a shift from content-based teaching to process-based teaching, where you are more concerned with *how* your learner is doing things rather than *what* they are doing. This sort of deep learning is sometimes called generative, or double loop, learning where the learner may learn some facts or skills, but particularly learns new ways of doing things, new ways of learning, or new ways of understanding themselves.

For example, the learner may be struggling to grasp what seems to you to be a very simple concept. 'I just don't seem to be able to get this,' your learner says to you. One way to tackle this as a teacher would be to tell the learner what they need to know, or perhaps to point the learner in the direction of suitable material encouraging them to learn this, and then checking out their learning when you next meet. In essence, this is content-based teaching. Process-based teaching would be to explore the reasons why your learner is having difficulties. This may need you as coach to focus much more on subtle cues, watching the learner carefully or listening to the message behind the words. The coach will probe to find out what it is that is missing, perhaps by asking what the learner needs to do in order to 'get this'. What could you do today that will help? The generative learning that is enabled by this approach is essential to continuing personal and professional development. The current speed of change, and overload of information demands that the adult professional learner develops deeper skills and attitudes of wisdom and decision making.

Flaherty suggests that there are five principles to coaching.[1] Of these five, he labels the relationship between coach and learner as the first and most important principle. The relationship or alliance is the background for all coaching, and must be one in which there is mutual respect, trust, and freedom of expression. The other four principles are pragmatism – an outcome focus with continual correction based on feedback; 'two track' – Flaherty's shorthand describing both the work coaches do with clients and the ongoing work coaches do with themselves; sensitivity to our learners' commitments, remembering they are already in the middle of their lives, with responsibilities and concerns outside their learning; and finally, remembering that techniques on their own don't work – challenging the routine way of applying techniques and remembering that our learners may resent it when techniques are applied to them.

So you as coach are a tool for the client. Your knowledge and methods of teaching are powerful tools. The learner, when he or she first comes to you, is rather like a block of marble, and the tools you have can be very effective in shaping that marble to becoming a perfect piece of sculpture, but only if they are applied at the right places. It is the learner's job to tell you where to apply them.

It follows that the designing of the alliance you have with your learner is fundamental to the success of your coaching. There are two main parts to this. First it is important to set up the alliance formally, exploring certain aspects with your learner right at the beginning. Second, it is essential to realise that the alliance is an ongoing process where you as coach and your learner evaluate the success of what is happening, adjusting what you are doing depending on the effect this is having. This may involve your learner asking you things, revealing what has worked and what has not worked, and also requires you to ask your learner questions about how you are doing.

Examples of questions to ask your learner are:

- How do you want to use me as your coach?
- What is working?

Questions to ask yourself are:

- What is working?
- Am I being used appropriately as a coach?

Setting up the alliance

It is always a good idea to start any one-to-one coaching relationship with a longer session – the intake session – to explore the way in which you will be working together and to get to know each other. The design of the alliance that you will have with your learner will be a major part of this intake session. It is here that your learner will discover what they can expect from you as their coach. It is here too that you as coach can set some of the boundaries and expectations you will have of your learner as coachee. You can explore with your learner some of the logistics that will make up the coaching relationship. It is a good idea to set some of these down in writing as a form of contract with your learner. By doing this you provide formal boundaries which aid safety and security. It also gives a factual basis for review as the relationship develops.

It is up to you to decide what you want to put in a contract. Our preference is to have a section on what the learner can expect from you as trainer or coach, the sort of processes which can happen and the actual structure of what to expect from formal teaching sessions. Some examples of the sort of things a contract might cover are included below.

Example of coach–coachee contract

I _____ am committed to creating a coaching alliance with .... (you as coach) .... This alliance will support me as I clarify and realise my goals and aspirations.

I want to work with you as coach to shape the coaching relationship to best meet my needs as learner by:

- clarifying what really matters to me
- learning about what helps me get on and do things
- identifying plans of action
- identifying key learning needs.

To do this, I want you as coach to:

- ask me honest and thoughtful questions
- challenge me by asking powerful questions
- help me commit to actions
- hold me accountable for those commitments
- help me forge a powerful working relationship.

I, as the learner, agree to:

- an initial intake that will last between one and two hours
- weekly tutorial sessions which will last at least one-and-a-half hours
- reschedule learning sessions no less than two days in advance
- regular reviews of the content and process of the coaching.

Your coach agrees to hold the content of our coaching sessions entirely confidential, as far as is permissible by law.

This is not a contract in the legal sense of the word but more a statement of the framework of the agreement you and your learner will have. It is a good idea to go through the contract point by point explaining to your learner what your expectations will be regarding the relationship. For example, regarding confidentiality in the agreement, it is worth clarifying exactly what you mean by this. If other members of your team are helping with the training, what sort of things will you be sharing with them? If you have a line manager or somebody you are expected to share aspects of the training with, what sort of things will you be sharing with them? Remember too that you may need to share difficult issues with your own coach or mentor; indeed you are entitled to such support, so you have to think how you will do that sharing – will it be nameless? What will your learner think of you sharing issues which they could possibly think put them in a bad light?

As well as agreeing how you will work together, it is equally important to state what coaching is not and what you are not prepared to engage with. This will vary from learner to learner and situation to situation. Generally coaches in a learning environment will not become involved in personal or psychological counselling, they will not engage in psychoanalysis, nor will they issue guidelines on right and wrong, unless it is very clear that the person they are working with is about to do something dangerous, illegal or totally unacceptable. Again a written description of what coaching is can be very helpful.

Example of an information sheet about coaching

Coaching is a designed alliance between a coach and a client which focuses on the aspirations of the client in order to enhance their personal and professional life. The client defines the agenda and the method of working, with the aim of creating balance, developing strategies and solutions, and creating choice. Coaching can work alongside other methods of training and teaching.

Coaching:

- is a journey with a guide who is curious and non-judgemental; a journey where you are given space to be and to think and to create the solution that fits for you
- is a bit like driving a car in the rain. The coach is the windscreen wipers clearing the screen so that you can concentrate on where you are going and how you are going to get there
- is a process of change which enables you to define what it is you really want, and then to make your desired future your achieved and enjoyable present
- is a practical, outcome-focused way of working
- is challenging and requires commitment
- recognises you as a resourceful and intact individual who has a unique set of values and beliefs which underpin how you perceive and behave in the world.

Coaching is not:

- giving advice or the right answers
- psychoanalytical
- counselling
- fixing or mending you.

Coaching does this by working in agreed sessions in order to define clear relevant and achievable goals. The coach may use a variety of techniques:

- support, encouragement and challenge
- reframing, metaphor, reflection and facilitation

- powerful questions
- working with values and beliefs.

Record keeping

Another aspect to consider as you design your alliance, is what sort of notes of your training sessions you will be keeping. This is something to share with your learner, and not just to share but also agree what can be jotted down for posterity. How safe will you keep your records? What will happen to them when your learner leaves? What sort of record keeping suits you? Are you going to keep detailed notes, or just jot down the headings, and then spend time thinking about them later?

Some coaches suggest that it is the duty of the coachee to keep the records, as the relationship is learner centred, and by keeping your own records, you, as coach, are deciding what is important. That is one point of view — generally it would be wise to keep some note of what you have discussed.

Getting to know each other

The basics

Having agreed how you are going to work together, it is now important in that first session to really get to know the person you are going to be learning with. There are obviously plenty of ways of doing this. One is to explore your learner's curriculum vitae (CV) with them, not just thinking about what they have done but also why they have done it and the positives and negatives of each appointment. It is also interesting to look at what they have not done — why didn't they pursue something that seemed so important at one stage of their life? You may share your own CV, or just talk a little about your life and what is important to you, let them know some of your highs and lows. The feedback we have received from our coachees is that presenting a human face is crucial to establishing trust and early effective working. It gives permission to the learner to be human and to admit areas of challenge. Though it may seem quite formal, it is also good practice to note down some key things about the learner. You would want to find out the following things:

- Their name and address, home and mobile phone, and email address.
- Their date of birth.

- What are significant things about their family?
- Who are their friends and significant others?
- Do they have special dates and anniversaries that are important to them?
- How do they spend their time when they are not at work?
- What are their hobbies and interests?

Some of these questions may seem obvious, but they are not always explored. We recently came across a learner who had failed after a year's professional apprenticeship. The trainer had no idea about his personal life or professional history, why he came to be where he was. Getting to know the person you are going to be working with is vital in any professional apprenticeship model of learning

It is also important to discover what drives and motivates the learner. You can get some of this information from doing more formal questionnaires such as learning styles, a Myers-Briggs Type Indicator (MBTI), or by looking at their meta-programmes (see Chapter 7), and it may be right to do this some time during their time with you. At the start, however, it is more appropriate to get a feeling for what drives the learning in your coachee, informally. Remember it is likely that the learner will not have been asked these sorts of questions before; indeed they themselves may never have even thought about what motivates them. The questions are best framed around statements such as: 'I want to understand how you work at your best so that we can really build on this in our time together.'

Where are you now? The wheel of life

Another useful area to explore at this early stage is the wheel of life. This is explained in more detail in Chapter 6, on tools and techniques. Essentially it is a way of looking at eight key areas in your learner's life, determining how important they are to your learner at this particular time of their life. Doing this now can help your learner to identify some of the key areas that they may want to address with you. It may well be, for example, that relationships in general do not score particularly high with your learner. Though clearly the relationship you have with your learner is not therapeutic, it may be appropriate to have a feel for issues outside the learning environment that might impact on the way they learn. The wheel of life is a way of helping you and your learner to be aware of some of these difficulties. It may well be that your learner excels in one of the areas. Why should that be? Are there strategies that they can get from that achievement that they can use towards successful learning? Or are there features about some of their less successful areas which could impact on and interfere with their learning?

Beliefs and values

One more thing to explore right at the beginning, is something about your learner's values and beliefs. Aspects of values and beliefs are covered in Chapter 8. Clearly these are things that will come up repeatedly during your time together, as these are core features of who we are. However, exploring this right at the beginning sets the tone of how your learning sessions may proceed. Getting to values and beliefs can sometimes be difficult. Questions that might help your coachee to think about this could be something like what issues really fire your learner, or what drives them really crazy. A list of value words that they can choose from can point them in the right direction too. In the end you can help your learner discover the top four or five values that really matter to them more than anything else. At a later session you may even choose to help your learner explore a hierarchy of these values. And you may also at some time want to think about hidden values, values which are important to your learner but which they find difficult to explore, or may not even notice.

Your learner's expectations

This is also the time to clarify what the learner can expect from you as coach. What is your side of the bargain going to be?
   Examples of questions that might move your learner forward are:

- How do you want to use me as your coach?
- What help do you need to become motivated?
- Do you want me to hold you accountable for actions we have agreed on?

Questions like these help your learner to focus on themselves as the instigator of actions in the relationship. This can certainly help develop a client-centred agenda, and you may want to raise questions like this again and again as the training progresses.

Primary focus

The final thing to think about at the intake session is what sort of areas your learner wants to deal with first. What will be the primary focus of the first few sessions? There may well be a curriculum that you have to follow as trainer, but there will be areas to explore first, so you and your learner need to work out together what these areas should be. In a client-focused agenda it is the client or learner who will set that agenda, though you as coach may well have useful tools for them.

Maintaining the alliance

Rapport

Rapport is the foundation of the relationship between you as coach and your learner. Getting good rapport with your learner at the start of coaching is really important. It is a good idea to remember though that every time you have contact with your learner you need to rebuild rapport.

So what is rapport? There are many ways of looking at this; one is to think of rapport as the state where there is an agreed, though often implicit, acceptance of issues of common concern. Two people can develop a feeling about the other within minutes or even seconds of first encounter. At interview, for example, the panel will often have judged a candidate before they sit down, and then use the interview to justify any initial decision. It is important to recognise our ability to discount others, for whatever reason, when we first meet them. Recognising this enables us to think about our own state, or internal feelings, so that we can accept other people, warts and all. You can often do this quite simply by spending a few minutes before meeting up with your learner to think about how you want to be as a coach. One effective way is to set your intent before you begin any coaching session. What sort of coach do you intend to be this time? Is this the time when you are going to hold back on what you say allowing your learner to speak more? Are you going to resist giving answers to questions this time? This short preparatory time looking at the process of your learning session rather than its content can pay dividends.

The second key component of developing rapport is to acknowledge the importance of both verbal and non-verbal communication. Mehrabian's work of 1981 showed that if your words and body language are inconsistent, then much more weight will be given to the body language than to the words.[2] Being congruent in words and actions is essential to good rapport – this is discussed in more depth under logical levels in Chapter 5. Another important area here is to have good but appropriate eye contact, remembering that there are cultural differences in the way people look at each other. A further useful ploy is to consider matching the postures and gestures of your learner, so, for example, if they are sitting cross-legged, matching them by sitting cross-legged yourself acknowledges their feelings in your posture. You can also match the voice patterns of your learner, such as the tempo of their speech, the pauses they make, or the sort of language they are using. Matching is powerful, but done to excess is just mimicking.

Another vital part of good rapport is to listen to what your learner is saying by actually hearing what they are saying. Again, though the words are important, deep listening comes from recognising the feelings and emotions behind those words. This sort of listening takes a lot of practice. It relies heavily on your intuition. It relies on you picking up on very small stimuli from your learner, on recognising what is both spoken and unspoken, and on you being keenly tuned to your own senses and how they are responding, and then acting on what you feel. It relies on listening not just to the words, but to the spaces between those words, the way words are phrased as metaphors, and is always deeply respectful and accepting of the learner. The questions that come from deep listening are skilful, focused, based on the learner's agenda, and never stray into advice giving.

Feedback

There has been a lot of talk in this chapter about there being an alliance between you as coach and the learner. It is important to remember it is an alliance and that you have your side as well. How are you going to assess your coaching skills? How are you going to keep your coaching alive and centred around the needs of the learner? How are you going to get feedback from your learner about what you're doing as coach? What are you going to do if the relationship between the two of you isn't going the way you think it ought to? All these require both feedback from the learner to you, and also self-awareness and reflection on what you yourself are doing. You need to assess what you're doing and how you're doing it, and then you need to think about what your intended outcomes are. How can you plan to move from what you are doing now to what you would like to be doing? It is important to let the coachee know that you will be constantly reviewing your own performance, and that you will be asking them for feedback so that you can make the relationship maximally worthwhile for their development. Recording coaching sessions either using video or audio is really helpful for you as a coach. It is vital to get consent from the learner first, and to explain to them who you will share the recordings with, how you will keep the recordings secure and how and when you will dispose of them.

As a coach you too need your supervision, mentoring, coaching or support. It is likely that your organisation will have developed some system for this to take place. It may be you have one-to-one coaching yourself. Or perhaps there will be some form of workshop to support you. Or maybe you will invest in some sort of co-coaching scheme where you and a colleague work together to support each other. However you do it, it is important you *do* do it. Training using coaching techniques is demanding. It requires preparation, action and reflection. This reflection is best done with someone else, a person who you can trust to give you feedback that will really enhance the way you work. The reward for you is that the process of training becomes a generative learning process for yourself that is challenging, exciting and fun.

References

1   Flaherty J (1998) *Coaching, Evoking Excellence in Others*. Butterworth-Heinemann, Oxford.

2   Mehrabian A (1981). *Silent Messages: implicit communication of emotions and attitudes*. Wadsworth, Belmont, CA.

4

What do you want . . . and how will you get it?

There are only 24 hours in a day, 168 hours in a week, 8760 hours in a year. There are easily as many things to learn. How do *you* choose what you want to do? How you know what is important enough for you to do something about today? Do you choose or does life just happen to you?

Every time we say yes to something we are saying no to something else. With every minute we are voting with our time. By reading this book you have voted to give time to personal and professional learning. There are many other ways you could spend this time. We suspect that you could generate a fascinating list of alternatives . . . don't . . . stick with it!

We are going to look at strategies for deciding what you really want, how to get there, how to recognise it when you are there and how to choose how much time and energy you will spend getting there.

Outcome versus problem frame

We live in a culture which is heavily aligned to problem solving, to looking for what isn't working, to find a solution or even someone to blame. The impact of this in education is so often demotivating and stifling. The price paid by the individual and the organisation is that they don't notice what is working, and they forget to consider what it is they actually want. In addition, if they do consider what they want it tends to have an 'away from' focus (I don't want something) rather than a 'towards' (I want this other thing) motivation.

Let us consider two possible frames for problem solving, the problem frame and the outcome frame.

Exercise

Consider a problem of medium severity in your life and ask the following questions:

Problem frame
- What is the problem?
- How long have you had it?
- Whose fault is it?
- What is the worst thing about it?
- Why haven't you solved it?

Stop and check out with yourself. How do you feel? How are you going to sort it out?

Now for the same issue ask these questions:

Outcome frame
- What do you want?
- When you have that, what will that do for you/give you?
- How will you know when you've got it?
- What resources do you have already that will help you?
- What is something similar that you did manage to do?
- What is the next step?

Now how do you feel? It is likely that these questions were harder to answer. It is also likely that a solution started to present itself and that you are feeling more positive.

Think about this when a learner presents you with a problem or an issue? For example a learner is very anxious about giving an opinion to a client for fear that they may be wrong. Compare and contrast the impact of the types of questions.

Problem frame	**Outcome frame**
What is the problem?	*What do you want?*
I feel very anxious	To feel OK expressing my views
How long has this been an issue?	*And what will that give you?*
For ever, since school.	More confidence, better rapport
What are you going to do?	*What is the first step to this?*
Try not to feel anxious.	Trying to see it from their
viewpoint.	

The outcome questions progress and gain a natural momentum which can be developed.

Each frame has different consequences. Many learners are habituated to their problems and deficiencies. They focus on what they perceive that they are doing badly. They focus on the detail of the problem, and their motivation is to escape from it (away from it). It is harder to be creative about finding solutions in the problem frame.

A consequence of using an outcome frame is that the focus changes from being 'away from' the problem, to moving towards a positive outcome. Learners can begin to create a future that they want. For some people this can be a new and threatening way of thinking. They may never have been asked or indeed considered for themselves, 'What do I actually want?' It is incredibly important to pace your learner here. The transition from staying immersed in the familiar problem, to opening and creating the future you want implies change. That can be scary. The message must be that the learner can change if *they* want to, and only when they know what it is they really want. The coach moves gently at the learner's pace without expectation or judgement. Implicit in this is the notion that the learner has choice. Contrast this to the didactic school of education which reverberates with statements such as 'what you need to know is this, and the way to do it is that.'

By using an outcome frame the coach promotes:

- an internally driven search
- a focus to a desired positive outcome
- an expectation that the learner is responsible for their learning
- an explicit goal
- the notion that the learner is resourceful and capable
- the notion of reviewing and marking success as steps are taken
- a foundation for further clarification, exploration and change.

These dovetail beautifully with the principles of adult self-directed learning. These are that adults are self-directed with a wealth of past experience, and that adults learn better experientially when there is a clear purpose and focus for the learning. Carl Rogers summarised these principles in his comment, 'The purpose of adult education is to help them to learn, not to teach them all they know and so stop them from carrying on learning.'[1]

Let us now consider how we refine what it is we want, so that we actually achieve it.

Creating a well-formed outcome

How do we get a successful outcome, for ourselves personally or professionally, or as an organisation? This is a common theme in management consultancy, in personal coaching and in cognitive behavioural therapies. The many models used often overlap. We will modify and apply the neuro-linguistic programming model of well-formed outcomes – see, for example, O'Connor, 2001 – and demonstrate how these can be used in a learning situation.[2]

What do you want?

This is one of the most powerful questions that we can ask ourselves or others. The more specific we can be, the more likely we are to get it. In a learning situation our needs are commonly defined in terms of:

- *Skills and behaviours*: to spell better, to consult more effectively, etc.
- *States*: to be more confident, to be more relaxed, etc.
- *Purpose*: to be clearer about understanding ourselves and others, to have a sense of direction.

There are four key areas to consider in creating a well-formed outcome:

- The 'want' stated in the positive.
- The success criteria.
- The appropriateness of the 'want' to you.
- The gains from the current way of doing things.

What do you want . . . stated in the positive

Many of us are surprised when we are asked what we actually want. Our natural response is often to state what we don't want. For example in a learning–coaching environment we often hear comments like 'I don't want to fail', 'I don't want to look stupid or show myself up', 'I don't want to spend forever doing this', 'I don't want to let this or that person down'.

By focusing on what is not wanted the learner runs the risk of disappearing down a black hole of anxiety where they do more of the same. You cannot think about what you don't want without thinking about it first. The classic example is 'don't think of a blue tree . . .'. You first have to see the blue tree to then not think about it. Our brains are programmed to the positive, and must think of the object before not thinking of it. So here is how we make the most of this: we ask, 'What do you want?' instead. And then, 'What will that give you?' Or 'What would having that do for you?' In this way we cycle upwards until the intention is stated in the positive.

Example

A learner is anxious about explaining something in a presentation because last time he got very flustered when asked some awkward questions.

Coach: What do you want?
Coachee: I don't want to look stupid.
Coach: What do you want instead?
Coachee: Well I want to look as if I know what I am talking about . . . even if I don't!
Coach: And what is important about looking as if you know what you are talking about?
Coachee: I will feel more confident.
Coach: And what will 'feel more confident' do for you?
Coachee: I'll be more relaxed and probably do a better job.
Coach: And what will you get out of that?
Coachee: I'll feel I've done my best, I'll be interested in what's going on . . .
I'll feel good and may want to do more!
Coach: So what is it you actually want?
Coachee: I want to be able to be relaxed and confident even if I don't know all the answers.

Now *there* is something constructive and positive to work with!

Another way of looking at this is to consider the purpose or the intention behind the 'want':

Ultimate purpose	*Example*
What is important about this?	To be myself
What will doing this enable you to do?	To learn
What will you get from this?	To know that I don't have to know it all
Purpose C	
What is important about this?	
What will doing this enable you to do?	
What will you get from this?	I will do a good job
Purpose B	
What is important about this?	
What will doing this enable you to do?	
What will you get from this?	Confidence, openness

Purpose A
What is important about this?
What will doing this enable you to do?   I will feel better
What will you get from this?   I will not be scared

Original 'want'/behaviour   *To feel less stupid*

Success criteria: how will you know when you've got what you want?

Outcomes, even when stated in the positive, are often vague and abstract. As in the previous example an outcome of being more confident will mean different things to different people. The focus now needs to be sharpened to creating a sensory-based behavioural description in order that the learner develops a clear image of how they will be. The analogy could be with manufacturing, where the success criteria or quality measures describe the wanted product. So, using the same example, now we ask:

- How will you know when you're more confident and relaxed?
- What will you be seeing?
- What will you be hearing?
- What will you be feeling?
- What will I see you doing when you've got this?

A more conversational approach to this is to ask what is known as the miracle question:

- Imagine that a miracle happens tonight while you are sleeping and when you wake you have suddenly become confident. Tell me what would be different now?

This works well when learners get stuck. Another approach is to ask them to think of someone that they admire who has the qualities that they want.

Appropriateness: can this be started and maintained by you?

This is the next step, the allowing of what has to be done.

Many learners give undue emphasis to outside constraints, they leave the outcomes in other people's hands and so set up a self-fulfilling prophecy of failure. We hear this in comments such as, 'Well, if only he would do this then I could do that' or, 'There are too many other things I'm supposed to be learning, exams don't test the right stuff anyway so I'm not going to bother.' Alternatively the learner may feel muddled about whether this is really them, comments such 'yes, well, on the one hand, yet on the other ...' or even, 'yes but ...' These comments suggest incongruence. The learner is not totally aligned with the idea – maybe it conflicts with one of their fundamental beliefs or values – maybe they think they *should* want this, but really they don't. We can all recognise incongruence. The classic example is opening a gift that you really don't like, from a well-intentioned friend, and having to hide your first reaction, saying something positive and thank you as if you mean it! *That* is the feeling of incongruence.

This is where we re-emphasise that this is the learner's outcome that they want for themselves and we ask about:

Internal ecology ... is this congruent for the learner?

- How does having this outcome honour the things that are really important to you, your values?
- How will this fit in with the rest of you and your life?
- Is it worth the time and energy to achieve this?

There are three areas to consider here:

- *Beliefs*:
    - do you want to achieve this outcome?
    - can you achieve this outcome?

If the answer is no then we ask:

    - what is it that you do want?

And then:

    - what is stopping you?
    - what do you need instead?

- *Context*:
    - when and with whom do you want this?
    - when and with whom do you not want this?
    - how long for?

- *Resources:*
    - what resources/skills do you already have that will help?
    - where have you done something similar?

By considering these areas, the learner can become much clearer on what they really want.

Gains from current behaviour

We often reject change for fear of the consequences of losing something else or becoming something else. We hear this in phrases such as 'better the devil you know', and 'mustn't throw the baby out with the bath water'. The secret of successful change and development is to know what you already have and to keep those bits that are valuable to you.

So it is important to take stock of what you are doing now and to actively choose to keep the bits you want. In doing this, the coach acknowledges that all behaviour has a purpose and that it serves the learner in some way, otherwise they wouldn't be doing it. If we believe that people are doing the best that they can at the time – given the choices available to them – then we can remain open, non-judgemental, interested and focused on what is best for the learner right now.

Openly acknowledging with the learner that we all do things for a reason, purposefully, is a powerful tool to use. It is honouring and respectful of where they are now. It does not seek to judge or assume a coach-delivered solution. It enables learner and coach to get curious about behaviour.

Example

Continuing with our first example, our session would continue:

Coach: We all do things for a reason; you have been doing this for a while because it serves you in some way. What do you get out of your present behaviour that you want to keep?
Coachee: Well, I suppose I don't come across as being arrogant.
Coach: Is that important to you?
Coachee: Yes.
Coach: What is not being arrogant?
Coachee: It is being respectful and tolerant.
Coach: So, as you achieve your goal of becoming more confident it is important for you to demonstrate your respect and tolerance?
Coachee: Yes.

Other questions that will access this information are:

- What will you gain/lose by achieving this outcome?
- What will you lose/gain by staying the same?

The learner has now taken the first most important steps to achieving what they want.

In summary, taking the time to consider these questions is the foundation of a successful outcome (see Figure 4.1). By working through the stages, the learner creates a detailed and compelling picture of what he or she wants. Confidence *and* capability increase as skills and resources that already existed are transferred, and there is a deep sense of congruency and self-worth for successful achievement. The most important steps have now been achieved. It becomes easy to move into the 'what has to be done', which is the first step, and actually planning and doing something.

Taking a learner through this process demonstrates the importance of choice and personal responsibility for learning and personal development.

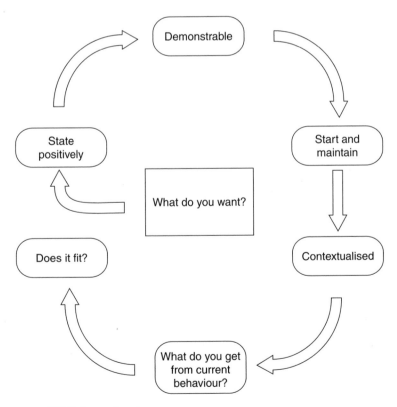

Figure 4.1   Well-formed outcome.

Learners who do this are more likely to complete tasks, to take less time over them and to be open to continuous review and development. They start to look at the detail of excellence, and they get curious about the specifics of how they can be what they want to be.

Creating the future

This is an extension of developing the success criteria for an outcome. It is a way of using that image to generalise any change to future situations and contexts. Specifically it allows the learner to test how they can be in the future. This process of mental rehearsal is used widely by sportsmen and presenters. It is the natural resource of a creative mind that is free to experiment. In teaching terms this is the precursor to role play. It is the internal representation of how the future will be. It can only be done once there is a well-formed outcome. The learner also needs to set an intent for how they want to be and behave.

Exercise

Think of a specific situation that is coming up in any part of your life where you want to be resourceful.

In your mind's eye create a movie screen and see and hear yourself in the picture in that situation in the future.

Run the movie and notice what happens.

You may run several different versions, make any adjustments that are necessary.

Run the movie and again notice what happens.

Now step into the movie and really get into yourself in that movie. Live the experience as it actually is. Feel what you feel, see what you see, and hear what you hear.

Step out of the movie and let go.

Think of an image or sound that will act as trigger for you when you step into this situation in the future and use that as an anchor that will help you remember how it is to be this person.

Procrastination

A most human habit! Most of us do this, in fact we can spend as much time and energy putting off a task as actually doing it. So, all these fine words about creating a successful outcome can at times feel fruitless. Your learner will choose to make a change, all will look rosy and positive but then ... nothing happens. The coach, coming from a position of curiosity with the presupposition that behaviour is purposeful, can hold a mirror up to the learner.

The coach will have the learner notice what they are procrastinating about and will ask questions such as:

- How is delaying helping you (there may be a very valid reason ... needing more information, a change in circumstances)?
- How much time/energy are you spending avoiding this?
- What is realistic?
- What is stopping you?
- What would happen if you achieved this?
- How are you approaching this? What other perspective could you take?
- How could this be easy or fun?

Here is an example of how this works in practice. A learner's desired outcome was to have two hours of focused purposeful reading a week. After two months, despite allocated study time, he still claimed that he never had time to do this. When asked how much time he was spending avoiding reading he laughed and said, 'I don't know but quite a lot I suspect.' He agreed to keep a diary and track how he spent his study time over one week. He discovered that he spent hours scanning the internet for possible resources (including holiday destinations), flicking through books in the library, and drawing up tables for recording his learning so that he could remember it for exams. Looking at how he used his time enabled him to consider how he wanted to use his time and to choose a different strategy for his study time. He achieved his desired outcome.

Acknowledging and challenging procrastination is an important process for coach and learner. It results in re-evaluation, and enables blocks to progress to be removed or the outcome to be modified. Perhaps, more importantly, in the long term, the learner will become aware of the signs of procrastination for themselves. They will learn to ask themselves these questions, and so move themselves forward. This is a fundamental skill for self-directed autonomous learning.

Mapping the journey

When designing a project, it is common to draw up a plan which is often timed and will include resources that will be needed along the way. In the same way, it is very valuable to the learner who wants to achieve a successful outcome to have a plan of how they will be feeling at different stages along the way. The authors have found that learners who keep this visual representation, or map, at hand tend to be more resourceful and tolerant of themselves. They are also more likely to achieve their desired outcome. This is a useful tool for projecting into the future.

As always the best way to learn a new tool is to do it yourself!

Exercise

Think of a project you have just started or are thinking about – it could be anything from clearing out your desk, to building a boat.

Copy the list below and fill the sections in numerical order:

Take the time to really go there, see what you see, hear what you hear and feel what you feel. The more real you can make it the more value you will get from this.

1   How will you feel when you have completed the task?
2   How do you feel as you contemplate this project at the beginning?
3   How will you feel halfway through the project/change?
4   How will you feel one-quarter of the way through?
5   How will you feel three-quarters of the way through?

Present . . . . Desired
2   4   3   5   1

Working through this enables us to do several things. We are able to create a compelling future – the picture becomes more real and felt and so we are more likely to continue to work towards it. By acknowledging how we will feel *en route*, we allow ourselves to be human ('it's OK to feel like this'). We can tolerate these states better and put strategies in place that will help. We are less likely to become despondent and more likely to persevere and achieve our desired outcome.

Key learning points

It is always worth investing in defining what it is that we want as a coach and as a learner. By becoming focused we save time and energy and we find our own solutions and create the outcome that is right for us.

1 Frame the issues around outcome not problem.
2 State what you want in the positive.
3 Define your success criteria.
4 Check the appropriateness of this for you.
5 Keep the good bits of what you have now.

References

1 Rogers CR and Freiberg HJ (1994) *Freedom to Learn* (3e). Merrill/Macmillan, Columbus, OH.

2 O'Connor J (2001) *NLP Workbook, a Practical Guide to Achieving the Results you Want*. Thorsons, London.

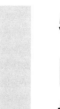

5

Feedback: the foundation for learning

- What do you believe about success, failure and feedback?
- What is your intention when you give feedback?
- What is your intention when you receive feedback?

Think carefully and honestly about these questions. Feedback is the foundation for learning. Your beliefs about success and failure and feedback will profoundly affect your learning. They will fundamentally affect your ability as a coach to open the door to learning for others.

For many, feedback is simply an acknowledgement of failure; it presupposes a hierarchical relationship where the person giving the feedback has the authority from knowing the best way. We learn early in life that failure is bad, even shameful. The language we use suggests that *we* are failures rather than we have failed at *doing* something. The result is that we learn to hide our failures, make excuses for them or ignore them. Feedback confronts this tendency, and so is commonly feared and avoided by both coachee and coach.

In reality, people are resourceful and creative, and they often succeed. They are not *failures*, even though they sometimes fail at *doing* something. The key to effective personal and professional development is to take the *learning* from the successes and the failures in life. The purpose of feedback is to feed forward from that learning so that we may have more choices in what we do.

There are many factors involved in giving effective feedback. We will look at the structure of how we give feedback and how we can take the learning from success and failure.

Learning from failure and learning from success

'Trial and error' and 'learning from our mistakes' ... these are phrases that we are used to hearing. They are phrases that remind us of our natural tendency to recall and analyse past failures. Not surprisingly a review is often called a 'post mortem'. Many people believe that this is the only way to learn. Traditional education was often based on such learning, where feedback was used to analyse failure. We fail exams, we fail to get the prize job, we fail to reach our potential. These failures are then often internalised and we consider *ourselves* failures. In contrast, how often do we formally analyse success? What was it that went well? How can we do that again and even better?

As we well know, there are few events in life entirely free from error, or totally devoid of success. To take the learning from both is the path to self-development and tolerance of self and others. Experience shows us that analysis in itself does not necessarily lead to learning with a resultant change in behaviour. We can analyse and 'understand' the reason behind a particular action, but that doesn't mean that we'll do it differently next time. We can't be the only ones to find ourselves groaning as we repeat the same old behaviour and find ourselves in the same situation exclaiming 'oh yes I remember this ...' It is easy to think of examples, the student who fails every exam first time, the girl who has repeated destructive personal relationships, the man who is always late to everything.

Table 5.1 The implications of analysing success and failure

Analysis of success	*Analysis of failure*
Can lead to:	**Can lead to:**
knowledge of causes of success	knowledge of causes of failure
understanding what went well	understanding what went wrong
Suggests:	**Suggests:**
things to repeat	things to avoid
things to do	things not to do
Can produce:	**Can produce:**
satisfaction	dissatisfaction
reassurance	uncertainty
confidence	lack of confidence
readiness to confront risk	wariness of risk
independence	dependence/suggestibility
warmth	anger
a willingness to cooperate	defensiveness
But may also encourage:	**But may also encourage:**
complacency	realism
arrogance	humility
reluctance to improve	determination to improve

The first stage in the learning can be the analyses of success or failure. Each has different implications and different value as can be seen in Table 5.1.

However, bearing in mind that the purpose of feedback is to help the coachee move from analyses to action, the coach must do more.

The coach asks:

- What is the learning in this?
- What is the gift here?
- What do you want to take forward?
- What do you want to let go of?

and

- How are you going to do that?
- What do you need in order to do that?
- What resources do you already have?
- What is the first step?
- When will you do that?

By asking these questions the coach acknowledges our humanness and our resourcefulness. The coach is tempting us forward to look at the structure of how we do things.

The structure of failure and success

For each of us success and failure has a pattern or a structure. Getting curious about and recognising the pattern is the first step to enabling flexibility and change . . . if that's what you want. The coach coming with an attitude of curiosity and non-judgement creates the space to look at this.

Exercise

We all have 'failure patterns', which are often unconscious and which keep us stuck even when we want to move on. Consider these: which ones apply to you?

- Not allowing yourself to dream
- Assuming change is hard work
- Being afraid of the unknown
- Setting unrealistic time frames

- Doubting your own ability
- Becoming cynical
- Believing that what you want can't happen
- Worrying about the effect of change on others
- Taking no for an answer.

Or maybe you sabotage success by:

- moving the goal posts – 'It's good to be a trainer but really I want to be an educational manager.'
- belittling your achievements (discounting) – 'Oh it was nothing ... anyone can do that.'
- not admitting what you really want – 'Things are just fine as they are ... then I don't have to face risk or disappointment.'

Patterns such as these often emerge and become apparent as the coachee progresses. These patterns can be ignored or they can be acknowledged and fed back to the coachee. The coach can hold a mirror up to the coachee so that they see their own reflection. Then the coach can use simple tools so that the frame around the mirror changes, and just as a landscape painting looks different with a different frame the coachee gains a new perspective. Not surprisingly, this is known as reframing, which is discussed in Chapter 6.

Example

- *I was never any good at statistics ... you never learnt a strategy for statistics ... you could if you wanted to.*
- *I really wanted that job, I feel a failure ... they gave the job to someone who they thought was better suited. What can you learn from that which will help you in future?*

Contrast this dialogue to the one that would have followed from the often used question 'Why?'. Why were you no good at statistics? Why do you think you are a failure? The 'why' question most commonly generates 'because' answers. It tends at best to lead to an 'I don't know' answer and at worst results in defensive explanations or justifications. Neither of these create real learning opportunities.

A more productive approach is to ask 'How' questions. This tends to move the learner forward and to create options based on what is practical and possible. Continuing with the previous examples:

- *You know that a basic knowledge of statistics is important . . . .*
  - *– How can you remind yourself of the basics?*
  - *– How can you ensure you have the information when you need it?*
  - *– How can you be most efficient in sorting this out?*
- *I wonder what you can learn from this experience that will help you.*
  - *– How did you prepare/feel/look?*
  - *– How could you have done it differently?*
  - *– And what will you do next time?*
  - *– And how will you remember to do* this?

Analysing success: It is interesting that when we look at success we more naturally ask 'how' rather than 'why?' We hear comments such as 'Wow how did you do that? rather than 'Wow, why did you do that?' In the same way that we have analysed the patterns of failure we can analyse the structure of success so that we can do more of it.

Exercise

Consider something that you have recently achieved. It can be a simple as you like – maybe you did those 20 minutes on the exercise bike three times last week, maybe you asked for feedback from your coachee about all your tutorials, or perhaps you didn't grumble at the children because the house was in a mess when you got home. Ask yourself the following questions:

- How did I set my goal?
- What sequence of things did I do, feel, hear and see that enabled this to happen?
- How do I know I succeeded? (think about internal and external measures)
- What was the difference that made the difference? What made it work this time?
- How can I do this more/again?
- What will I do now?

Imagine a feedback session based on these questions, looking at success. How will you feel? How will the coachee feel?

Logical levels

A useful idea to come from neurolinguistic programming is that of logical levels. It has particular relevance when we are considering feedback, as it points to where and how feedback is best given. The concept suggests that all of us have six levels of function – sometimes these all work together, and we feel congruent. At other times they fail to cooperate and we 'fall apart' and feel stressed, uncomfortable or sad.

The first level is the environment, where and when we do things, and who we do them with. Success may come if you are 'in the right place at the right time'. The second level is behaviour, what we do. This includes thoughts as well as actions. The third level is capability or skill, and describes how we do things. You can't see a person's skills, but only deduce it from their behaviour. The fourth level is about values and beliefs, why we do things – they give purpose and meaning to what we do (and are further discussed in Chapter 8 on values and beliefs). The fifth level is identity, who we are. This says something about the sort of person we are. The sixth and final level is beyond identity, and describes something about our connection with what is outside us, about ethics, religion and spirituality (Figure 5.1).

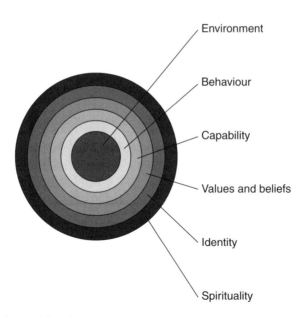

Figure 5.1   Logical levels.

These levels are not a hierarchy – they connect and interrelate and influence each other. You can get a feel for their meaning when you think about yourself as a *coach*.

Logical levels are a valuable tool in understanding situations and in deciding where and how to intervene. When we are giving feedback we are thinking about change and development. When we want change it is useful to think about at which logical level we are attempting it. As we progress up the hierarchy of levels the interventions are different.

As a coach we use logical levels to develop our skill in giving feedback.

- *Identity*: Who am I as a I give feedback? Am I equal to the learner?
- *Beliefs and values*: What do I believe about feedback? What is important to me?
- *Capability*: What skills do I have? How can I improve my skills?
- *Behaviour*: What do I actually do when I give feedback?
- *Environment*: What is the best place/time to give feedback?

The coach giving feedback believes that the learner is bigger than their behaviour, that the learner themself is not a failure.

Giving feedback using logical levels – 'behaviour not identity'

It is a well-recognised premise that 'good feedback' is about behaviour, not about identity. We say 'I notice that you find it difficult to find things in your room' rather than 'you are such a messy individual'. Using logical levels we can also help the learner unpick what factors are important about environment and where there are skills to be developed or behaviours to be changed.

In the coaching model of learning and development it is also possible to raise the issues of belief and identity. Working at this levels requires an established relationship of trust and non-judgment. We do not assume or name what we perceive to be a belief or identity issue, nor do we presume to change it. We can, however, reflect and ask questions such as:

- I wonder what you believe about your colleagues when you chair a meeting with them.
- Who are you when you do this?

Your intention and the purpose of feedback

The purpose of feedback is to:

- create a foundation for future success
- discover the learning in an experience
- recognise that it's OK to be human.

How often do we hold this in our mind and heart as we plan and deliver our feedback? How often when you have been the receiver of feedback have you sensed this purpose?

Your intention is what most profoundly affects how you give feedback and how your feedback is received and used. Your intention will be based on what you perceive is the purpose and value of giving feedback. We can all recall times when feedback was not as great as it could have been: that hurried chat in the corridor, the in-depth analysis littered with pearls of wisdom from you, the tempered 'telling off' masked as a learning opportunity. Some of what makes these less fruitful experiences are to do with the time and place. Fundamentally though it is about the state that the giver and receiver are in and what the primary intention is.

Exercise

Take two minutes for each scenario.

Think of a time when you felt that you:

- gave really good feedback
- gave bad feedback
- really benefited from feedback that was given to you
- rejected, ignored or felt angry about feedback that was given to you.

These times could be in a formal teaching situation or informally talking to a friend, your partner or your child. If you can't think of an example, consider when you have seen someone else in that situation, put yourself in their shoes and imagine how it was for them.

You may find it helpful to keep notes.

For each scenario ask yourself:

- How were you feeling?
- What did you see?

- What would the other person have seen about you?
- How did your voice sound?
- What was the dialogue in your head about?
- What did you think/believe about yourself?
- What did you think/believe about the other person?
- What was your intention?

Sometimes the answers can be surprising . . . what have you discovered about yourself?

Setting intent is a very powerful thing to do. Shaman healers will tell you that setting their intent is the most important factor in their work. You can set intent very simply by saying, 'My intention is to . . .', 'I intend to . . .'

The purpose of feedback is to enable the receiver to be the best that they can be by creating options and choice for the future.

Hold this purpose in your mind and set your intent as you prepare for your next feedback session. Notice the difference it makes.

Asking permission or not

Asking permission demonstrates that you are sensitive to the coachee. It demonstrates the purpose of giving feedback – that it is for their learning. It is not about you being better and having the right answer. Of course, if you are going to ask permission you have to respect the coachee's wishes. If you ask, 'Can I give you some feedback on the way you handled that phone call' and your coachee says, 'I'd rather you didn't', then it's best not continue to pursue it at that stage. Another way of asking permission is to first highlight an issue as a statement of fact. For example:

'I notice that you have new ideas and plans each week, but nothing seems to be happening. May I ask you what the resistance is to actually doing? Would you be willing to look at that?'

There will be times when you feel strongly that you have a duty to address certain behaviours. Under these circumstances do not ask permission. Here it is useful to be explicit about what you are going to do and what the purpose is. For example: 'I am going to give you some feedback about how I heard you handle that phone call. I think there is some important learning there.'

Safety and challenge

As educationalists we are already skilled in the art of giving feedback. We are aware of the importance of preparation, environment, timing and our own psychological state. We use such models as the feedback sandwich to give our feedback (see Chapter 7 on meta-programmes). How do these work in practice?

Just recall for a minute when you receive feedback ... how many times have you said aloud or in your head 'OK, OK just tell me what I did badly and how I can do it better'? How many times have you not even heard the successful bits, let alone taken time to reflect on them and consider how to develop those skills still further. And what do you hear and see from your learners when it is feedback time? When you use the feedback sandwich is it as effective as it could be?

The challenge for the person giving the feedback is to offer it in a way in which it can be heard. For any peak performance there is a fine balance between the adrenaline of challenge and the confidence in existing skill. One way to do this is to also consider the mix between safety and challenge.

Generally we gain most from feedback when the balance is 75% safety and 25% challenge:

- 75% – what went well and why?
- 25% – what else might have worked?

What would be a stretch for the person to try next time? What is the growing edge for this person?

Notice the term stretch. This suggests something that is within reach with a little effort. It is not about reaching for the sky in one move. It is also one stretch – it is not about itemising 10 different new behaviours that they may like to try next time. Keeping it simple and focused ensures that you maintain their interest and the belief that this is possible. As this is repeated, the coachee will model themselves on you and will automatically start to look for the learning in an experience. The coachee will set their own 'challenges' or stretches ... and invariably they will be tougher and more relevant than any you could have set.

Observation and simple questions

Effective feedback uses facts and detail. It makes a deliberate search for the learning in an experience by helping the coachee to analyse the evidence. It is not a mind reading exercise. It is not about interpreting someone else's behaviour in the light of your own experience and beliefs. By looking at the structure of success and failure, feedback becomes about behaviour, not identity. The coachee will gradually start to reframe from 'I am a failure' to 'I didn't do that as well as I might, what do I want to do now?'

Stating fact and observation from a non-judgemental position, and asking simple questions are the most powerful tools of feedback. In an effort to appear gentle, the coach can ramble through a long presupposition about what may or may not have been the cause of the behaviour, and then ask such a complicated question that even she gets lost. Remember, the most powerful questions are the short ones. The coachee will need to think before responding, and there will be the learning.

Example

Consider a medical example, about giving feedback after watching a doctor in training giving antibiotics to a teenager for a one-day history of a sore throat (a situation where many realise that antibiotic pre-scriptions are of little use).

Option 1:
Coach: The issues around prescribing are so complex. There are obviously many factors involved including the fact that I am sitting in and watching you, which I understand will affect your behaviour at times, but I just wonder why did you give that 16-year-old antibiotics?
Coachee: Well I was running late, I thought that's what he wanted, he got them last time; I don't know . . .

These are all possible answers, which don't in themselves lead to learning for next time.

Option 2:
Coach: I notice you prescribed antibiotics. What other choices did you have?
Coachee: I could have not prescribed, I could have given a script to be dispensed in a couple of days if necessary . . .

These answers generate options which invite further questions such as, 'What would happen if you did that?' It is here that there is learning for the future.

There is no such thing as failure, only feedback.

What a statement! This is a presupposition taken from the applied psychology of neurolinguistic programming. A presupposition is not necessarily true; however, to function as if it were true can have a profound impact on behaviour. Just imagine if you went through life believing that there was no such thing as failure, only feedback .... . Remember those times in school, interviews and discussions with your partners. How often have you taken only what was negative from a feedback session, and left feeling worthless, a failure? How often has your heart sunk when someone taps you on the shoulder on a course and says, 'Can I just have a word about what you did just then?' How could your life have been different if you had been curious and interested in feedback, if you believed that there was no such thing as failure, only feedback in order to feed forward? The coach giving feedback believes that the coachee is bigger than their behaviour, that the coachee is not a failure.

Summary

These are some attributes that will enable you to give feedback that is really heard and that is really effective.

- *Setting a positive intent*: to help the receiver to be the best that they can be
- *An attitude of curiosity*: how did they do that? I wonder if that's part of something else? Where else might that happen?
- *Knowing that we each perceive the world in a different way*: neither is right or wrong, both perceptions can be useful.
- *Believing that feedback is about behaviour not identity*: it is about what they are doing not about who they are.
- *Believing that the person to whom you are giving feedback is bigger than their behaviour.*
- *Believing that it is better to have choice rather than no choice*: the gift of feedback is that it creates awareness of choice.
- *Being gentle* and *honest* – as opposed to being gentle or honest.
- *Framing the feedback around the stretch*: what might be their growing edge.
- *Keeping it short and simple.*
- *Working to acknowledge.*

6

Coaching tools

Some techniques really help the flow of coaching. We have chosen a selection of tools which we find really useful and which tend to move things along. None of these is an answer in itself, and there are other ways of getting the most from a coaching session. Likewise, there is no question of a session being poor because none of these has been used. It is important to remember too that the most important tool in coaching is yourself – you have a unique place in helping a learner learn and develop, and using your presence in a teaching session can make that learning even richer and deeper.

This is similar to the way you as a person have such an important part to play in any personal transaction. For example, Balint in 1957 wrote about the medical consultation in which the doctor himself or herself is often as important as the therapeutic intervention itself.[1] When you are being a coach to your learner, how you act or how you manage yourself can make an enormous difference to the teaching session itself. So how do you go about preparing yourself for a teaching session so that you are in the best possible frame to help your learner learn optimally? One helpful way to do this is to think about how you want your teaching session to go before you start. This is often called setting your intent. Spend five minutes before you meet your learner thinking about how you intend to be in this teaching session. Maybe you're the sort of teacher who likes to talk a lot, who likes to tell your learner how to do things. You might care to set an intent to spend more time listening and at a deeper level than usual. Perhaps you choose to set an intent to listen carefully to the words your learner uses, or to explore some of the non-verbal cues. Getting in the right frame before a teaching session will help the flow more than almost anything else. This is not just about getting the environment right or of having an hour or so of uninterrupted time; it is deciding how you want to be while coaching. This is closely related to developing the coaching alliance which is discussed elsewhere.

Accountability

Using a coaching frame for teaching and learning in itself sets up accountability. The trainer and learner together set up an alliance in which the learner can talk about things that work and do not work for him or her. This accountability is not just about task, though. It is helpful to also hold your learner accountable for the vision and process of learning, and for ways in which they can move their learning forward. It is helpful to talk about this way of working early in the relationship you have with your learner. You may care to check with them how they feel about being held accountable, and ask their permission to do so.

We often set our learners tasks to do in between supervisions. They may have not been able to do these for a variety of reasons. Maybe the tasks were too big. Perhaps the learner is busy with family life. Or maybe they just find it difficult to get down to the business in hand. Holding them accountable can help them do what they said they would do. Several questions are useful for the learner here, divided into questions related to the task and questions related to process.

Task questions:

- What are you going to do?
- By when will you do this?
- How will you and I both know you have done it?

Learning or process questions:

- Where are you playing helpless?
- Where are you being active as a learner?
- Which stretch is right for you now?
- How do you want to be as a learner?
- What do you need in order to be that learner?

Example

A learner has just had a tutorial with you. He has agreed that he will look further into some issues that have been discussed.

Coach: So what exactly are you going to do?
Coachee: I will follow up on the issues we have been discussing and let you know what I discover.
Coach: So exactly what is it you are going to do?

> *Coachee*: I will find out the commonest causes of what we have been discussing.
> *Coach*: And when will you have done this by?
> *Coachee*: I'll make sure I have done it by the next time we meet.
> *Coach*: And what is it you will be bringing to our supervision?
> *Coachee*: I will bring a list, and maybe some more detail.
> *Coach*: And is that something you would like me to hold you accountable for?
> *Coachee*: Yes, please.

Accountability is a key part of coaching; as mentioned above it is implicit in the relationship itself. It can however be overused. In particular, using it as the only means of moving a stuck learner forward may overlook the real reasons why they are finding progress difficult. Maybe there is something here about a limiting belief, and holding him accountable will not address that issue. Part of the skill of being a coach is to know when to hold the learner accountable, and when to explore other issues in their lives. Check out frequently how things are going, and how the questions you are using are helping the learning.

A repeated pattern of asking to be held accountable and then not achieving is a huge learning opportunity for the learner. It is your role as coach to be aware of this, to bring it into the open and to challenge the behaviour.

Acknowledgment

We are taught to give positive feedback to our learners – indeed giving feedback where things that could be changed are sandwiched between positive statements is a core part of training. Positive feedback is often given in the form of praise, 'I liked how you started that presentation', or in terms of factual behavioural comments, 'Your delivery was clear and the handouts user friendly.' These comments may make a learner feel approved of, liked or valued. It takes a wise and experienced learner to ask beyond this for the specifics, 'What particularly about my handouts was user friendly', or, 'What specifically did you think went well and why?' Praise focuses on the giver rather than the receiver, and tends to comment on behaviour, on what the person does. Praise encourages the learner to continue to seek the coach's approval rather than look at who they really are.

Acknowledgement, on the other hand, focuses on the learner and who they are, rather than what they have done. When acknowledging the learner, the coach points out something positive about who the learner really is, demonstrating a deep understanding of the learner and operating at the identity level (see logical levels, p. 46). The best way of illustrating the difference is through an example.

A learner may have had considerable difficulty with working with conflict. She finds it difficult to express her professional opinion. She wrestles with an internal dialogue on the one hand resisting the pressure, but on the other hand wanting to help. In the end she expresses her opinion. She discusses this with her coach. Her coach responds: 'Congratulations. That took courage, I know you have felt really uncomfortable doing this, and you now know that you can say what you really feel.' This is acknowledgement. It goes to where it is really heard, reinforces her growing edge and empowers her to keep growing. Another coach, who tends to praise, might respond: 'That was a good thing to do, I am proud of you for doing that.' This looks at behaviour, at what she did, and focuses on the trainer and what they are feeling.

The skilled coach also looks carefully at the effect acknowledgement has on the learner. If your acknowledgement is right on target, the effect on the learner can be profound, as it really speaks to them. Some learners may find true acknowledgment difficult to hear, as it is not always something they are used to. They may squirm or apologise or discount what you are saying. We are all very good at discounting acknowledgement when we hear it: 'oh, that's nothing', or 'just doing my job'. It may be useful for them to just hear what is said, and to be encouraged to just say 'thank you' after your acknowledgement.

Exercise

Be aware over the next few weeks of your natural tendency over giving positive feedback. Do you praise or acknowledge? Watch yourself with children, with colleagues, staff and learners. Notice the impact of your words on others.

Praise phrases:
- I'm proud of you.
- I'm pleased.
- That was good.
- I'm impressed.

Acknowledgement phrases:
- That took courage.
- Notice how it was this time with you stepping back for a moment?

- You really persevered, and look at the effect.
- What is it in you that enabled you to take that step? And how might you tap into that again?
- That was a stretch for you and you did it.

Balance wheel

The balance wheel (Figure 6.1) helps a learner explore and assess how things are in eight key areas in their life. You as trainer can decide what each segment represents. In our trainers' coaching practice in the South West of England we have chosen to highlight eight areas: health, continuing professional development (CPD), relationships at work, personal skills and resources, systems and tools, conflict management, time management and work/life balance. In mainstream coaching, the segments often look at work, health, personal growth, money, fun and recreation, friends and family, love and romance, and the environment (as in Figure 6.1). You and your learner may decide to choose your own categories.

The balance wheel is a snapshot – learners may find that it changes day by day or year by year. The eight sections in this wheel represent a balance. If the centre of the wheel is regarded as having a value of 0 and the outer edge 10, the learner ranks their level of satisfaction with each life area by drawing a straight or curved line to create a new outer edge. 0 means that

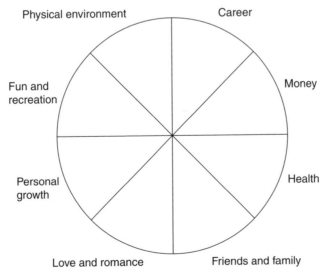

Figure 6.1   The balance wheel.

they aren't at all happy with that area right now, whereas a score of 10 means that they would find it difficult to think how this area could be improved. Using this tool, a learner can explore key values and beliefs, can think about parts of their life they are not paying proper attention to, and investigate where change could be most effective.

A learner may fill in the wheel as in Figure 6.2:

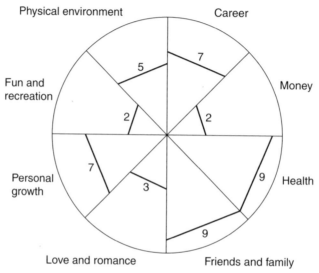

Figure 6.2   A completed balance wheel.

This wheel suggests a perception of a life currently not in balance. Health and family are going well, but there are some areas of discussion around romance, money and fun. Many questions can arise from this. How does the learner know that a segment has that score? What would it be like if that segment was to score 10 – or even 1? What is the difference between the two, and if the learner wants to make a change, what would need to be different? What would it take to make that move? What did the learner notice from doing the wheel? Who are you when everything is in balance? What do you want to change and how could you do that? What is the learner not paying attention to in their life right now? Is there a wedge which has most leverage, which if you changed could have an impact on other areas? For the trainer, there are no judgements to be made, just curiosity – once you start to judge, then you can no longer be curious.

Completing a balance wheel is not only a good way of starting a learner's year (see 'Designing the alliance' p. 15), it is also a good tool to use throughout the year, looking at change and progress. It also helps explore areas that are really important to a registrar, and helps you help them with attitudinal issues.

Bottom lining

People are great story tellers, indeed the narrative and case study are cornerstones of learning in medicine, law and other disciplines. Sometimes, however, the story can be a way of avoiding action. We can all be left wondering, just what was the point of that story, or where is it leading to? Bottom lining is the skill of brevity and succinctness by both coach and learner. It helps the learner clarify what the essence of the issue is. Bottom lining can be quite a shock for a learner when it first happens. It may be a good idea to warn the learner, right at the beginning of their time with you, that from time to time you may cut across the story to help them explore where the real issues are.

In case analysis or supervision, the learner may be explaining to you what happened when working with a client:

Example

Coachee: Mrs Smith came to see me again. I really don't know what her particular problem is, she seems to come and see me every week with the same sort of problem, one week it is this, the next it is that, and the next it is something completely different ...

Coach: So what do you think the bottom line really is here?

Coachee: I really do want to help people like Mrs Smith who seem to have multiple problems. There seem to be so many of them. I just don't seem to find a way of helping them.

Coach: So what is the real issue here?

Coachee: These people seem to swamp me, I feel so inadequate.

Coach: You feel so inadequate? That seems to be something really important. How would you like to work on that?

By bottom lining, you not only help the learner untangle what is really going on, but also make the best use of teaching time available. It is worth remembering also that bottom lining is a skill that you as coach can be using about the way you talk and relate to your learner. If you have a tendency to ramble around an issue, ask yourself 'what is the bottom line here?' and allow your learner to do the talking!

Some useful bottom lining questions include:

- What is the bottom line here?
- What is this about?

- What is at the heart of this?
- What value is being honoured or violated here?
- In a nutshell what is this about?
- What is the key point in this?

Challenging

People working in new areas often find certain things hard. This may be because of a genuine lack of knowledge and skills. Often, though, it is because the learner has self-imposed limits and beliefs about what they can and cannot do. Challenging asks the learner to extend themselves beyond what they think they can do. Good challenges stretch learners beyond what they are really capable of, so they may well react with surprise and disbelief. Yet the challenge itself indicates the belief the coach has in the learner and can be quite empowering. Often the learner will come back with a response indicating that they could not possibly do what you're asking, and suggest something less onerous. Equally the learner may come back with a challenge far harder than you would ever have set!

For example, the discussion may be centring on a learner's difficulty in keeping to time, so, for example, in the medical context, the coach may challenge the learner to make sure every consultation in the next surgery lasts no more than 10 minutes. 'I can't possibly do that!' replies your learner. 'So what would be a reasonable number?', 'I guess I could probably aim for half the consultations.', 'Have a go at that and then see how things are when we next meet.'

So the learner has set their own target which is certainly achievable, but also sets the level of challenge to be more than the learner might have done without the intervention.

It is helpful to consider challenging not just by setting a difficult task, but also by challenging the processes that are taking place during a learning session. This may show itself by inconsistencies between your learner's behaviour and the values that you know your learner has. Or your learner may behave in a particular way during the tutorial, which is not conducive to their learning or to the goals they have set. For example they may consistently be late for teaching sessions that have been planned for some time. There may be a real reason on one or two occasions, but repeated behaviour like this is worth challenging. The conversation went something like this with a learner:

Coach: I notice that you always arrive late for our sessions together, you appear hassled and it takes some 10 minutes for you to become focused.

Coachee: Oh yes, sorry, it happens all the time . . . I just get so involved with what I'm doing then someone asks me to do something and I try and squeeze that in too.

Coach: So how is this behaviour serving you?

Coachee: Well I suppose it's not me, it's others really, people think I'm nice and approachable and give of my time freely and it sort of works out that way, it doesn't seem right to say, 'I am on my way to a meeting and I need time to prepare.'

Coach: Oh? So what message are you giving?

Coachee: I'm not sure, something about where my priorities are, can't say no . . .

Coach: How would you like it to be?

Coachee: I'd like to stop feeling in a rush and sort of on overwhelm the whole time.

Coach: And when you're not in rush and not on overwhelm how is that?

Coachee: Clearer, calmer and more focused.

Coach: Is it important for you to have this in tutorials or meetings?

Coachee: Yes.

Coach: What is the first step?

And so on.

Forwarding the action

To some extent this is an amalgam of all coaching skills, and is the essence of what coaching is about, with an emphasis on moving the learner forward. A coach is forwarding the action when they are curious with their learner about what they want, the difference this will make for them and how they will know they are getting some of what they want. This is partly about helping the learner make plans, but is also about the coach helping the learner be curious about why they want that course of action, and to feel confident to explore new avenues and new ways of doing things.

This concept seems simple and obvious, but is in fact quite hard. It requires a combination of intuition, of knowing your learner well, occasionally stepping back and saying nothing, and at other times asking a powerful and insightful question which will help the learner see issues in a new way. You can notice when you are not forwarding the action with a learner, because the conversation appears more like chat and both parties are getting interested in detail rather than the essence of the story.

Asking what the bottom line of the story is might help when this happens. Other useful questions might be to ask 'what's next?' or 'what will get you started?', or even to say 'I'm curious to know what's going on here.' You may even choose to feed back to your learner what is going on in your mind about how you are feeling about the coaching session. It may be a bit blunt to say outright that you are bored, but you could certainly phrase that idea in a way that helps move the registrar forwards. You might care to think how you *could* phrase that.

Holding the learner's agenda

As a trainer you have a professional obligation to ensure that your learner reaches certain standards and capabilities. You will definitely have your own agenda, and frequently this and the learner's agenda are parallel. When using coaching as a form of training, however, it is really important to be *centred* on the learner's agenda. This is both a skill and a way of being. You have to let go of your opinions and judgements, following the learner's lead without knowing where the end will be. It means your attention must be wholly on the learner, and not on your agenda of how they should or should not be.

This does not mean you have to slavishly follow their agenda. There may be times when your mind is busy and occupied because of other things in your life. Something that comes up with a learner may trigger some ancient memory in you. You may find you are totally at odds with their agenda, perhaps for moral reasons. Or what they are saying may even be dangerous or risky. That's the time to stop and consider what is happening. The secret is to be in tune with yourself, to recognise when you are not congruent, and then to do something about it, maybe a pause, maybe you even need your tutorial on another day. You also need to be explicit about what *their* agenda is and think about where *your* boundaries lie.

This begs the question that both you and your learner know what the agenda really is. Is it about the doing of day-to-day issues and being held to account for these, or is it about exploring what the person you are working with really is about, what their values are, what makes them tick and what will help them in their continuing development?

Questions which might help hold you to your learner's agenda can include:

- Will this matter to you 10 years from now?
- How does this action match your values?
- What is really important to you?

A key strategy is to engage in deep listening. Deep listening is about hearing not only the words but also the messages behind the words. Clues to those messages come from the non-verbal communications you pick up. And there

	Known to self	Not known to self
Known to others	Arena *Open*	Blind spot *Feedback*
Not known to others	Facade *Sharing and self-disclosure*	Unknown *Exploration*

Figure 6.3 Johari window.

is more to it than that. There is something about picking up the energy of communication, using your intuition, and trusting your senses. Using all your antennae will enable you to work closely with your learner's agenda.

Much has been written about how to pick up non-verbal communication. Looking at posture, seeing small facial expressions, watching your learner fidget while they talk about something can help you decide whether or not they are being really congruent. One useful way of doing this is to think about the Johari window (Figure 6.3). Think about the way you communicate with others as being divided into four boxes. The first of these – the arena – considers what is known and open to both you and your learner. The second – the blind spot – describes things which are known to you but not to the learner. The third – the facade – considers things which are known to your learner but not to you. The fourth – the unknown – is about things which are not known to you or your learner. As coach, you can help your learner increase the size of their arena by helping them shrink the facade and the blind spot by a combination of self-disclosure and feedback. Working with the unknown can be useful, but can also be tricky and require considerable skill.

Inquiry

Setting an inquiry at the end of the coaching session is a bit like giving some homework. Unlike traditional homework, however, an inquiry works with the learner's agenda rather than that of the teacher. The inquiry will often consist of a powerful question coming from issues the learner has been wrestling with during the coaching session. The question can help the learner deepen their learning, so provoking further reflection. The learner can consider this question between sessions, seeing what occurs to him or her. It is important for the coach to make note of the inquiry so that it can be addressed at the next session.

Example

A learner found it very difficult to relax and was always filling her time with things to do. One training session revolved around how she would spend the time after her training year. The learner was talking about moving immediately into jobs yet remained uncertain about what direction she wanted to take in life. 'What is a pause for you? asks the coach. Reflection on this in the intervening weeks allowed the registrar to think of reasons why she needed to keep her life so full.

As with powerful questions, the elegance of an inquiry is both its simplicity and its depth, and the connection it makes with the learner's own agenda. Some examples of questions which might be inquiries include:

- What might happen?
- What keeps you going?
- What is it to be right?
- What is learning for you?
- Who are you becoming?
- What you assuming?
- What is pleasure?
- What will keep you on track?

Powerful questions

Questioning rather than telling is one of the key skills of learning through coaching. Socrates knew about this centuries ago. Powerful questions create new learning, increase clarity and discovery, and lead to greater creativity and insight. They encourage the learner to look in new directions and to explore new ways of seeing things.

They are usually deceptively simple and short, forcing the learner to answer from the heart. They are always open questions – that is, questions which cannot be answered yes or no. The way they are framed can help your learner in searching for the answer. Some questions may be provocative, encouraging the learner to become quite defensive when answering them. 'How did you expect to keep to time when working with people?' implies something the learner would find very difficult to do. Try and avoid questions that just seem to be gathering more and more data without really moving things forward.

The essence of powerful questioning is not to give your learner the answer. Many times the learner can find the answer within themselves and often surprise themself with the depth and quality of their understanding of an issue. It is possible to conduct a whole tutorial or supervision just using powerful questions, and it can be quite amazing the amount of ground covered.

Examples of powerful questions might include:

- So what do you really want?
- Where do we go from here?
- What does that say about you?
- How do you feel about it?
- What else?
- What will you take away from this?
- What will you do?
- Now what?
- Where do you go from here?

Though powerful questions are simple, the elegance is often in their timing. And sometimes the best questions come from your own intuition or hunch. It is sometimes worth blurting out what you are really feeling rather than analysing it first. It is also important to allow time and silence. A barrage of powerful questions one after the other is overwhelming and soon breaks rapport.

Framing and reframing

How you frame coaching sessions with your registrar can make a big impact on their learning. In much the same way as a picture frame can seem to change the colours and textures of a painting, so framing a tutorial can make big changes to learning. One example of this is to put a time frame around a session – the question 'We've got 10 minutes left in this tutorial, what would help you get the most out of that time?' (note, not 'what would you like to do?') can help focus your learner and you on what really needs to happen. You may also choose to use an outcome rather than problem frame, perhaps changing a 'problem case analysis' into an 'outcome-focused analysis'. Another useful frame is the 'as-if' frame, during which you help the learner imagine how it would be to have a particular skill or approach to work. You could phrase a question such as, 'I know you are not yet able to counsel effectively, but suppose for a minute you could, how would that feel …?' This allows the learner to see the world from a different angle, to try things on for size before actually getting there.

Reframing, on the other hand, provides your registrar with a different perspective on what is happening. By reframing, the coach takes information from the learner, telling it back in a different way, helping the learner see things in a new and constructive way.

Your learner may from time to time get stuck with a particular problem or way of working with clients. Every time the issue comes up, they travel down the same path with the same result. Sometimes when you are enmeshed in a problem it is difficult to see there may be other ways of doing things. As a coach, you can help the learner reframe the problem. For example, your learner may be having real problems settling down to preparing material for assessment.

Example

Coachee: I have been working on this for four weeks yet I seem no further forward.

To reframe, the coach steps back and helps the learner see the issue from a new perspective.

Coach: I remember when you started preparing for your assessment, you seemed quite excited and challenged by the new material.
Coachee: Yes, that's right.
Coach: So let's look at what you have learned in those four weeks.
Coachee: Well, come to think of it, I have learned how to organise my learning, and balance my time between work and home more.
Coach: That's great, is there anything else?
Coachee: Yes, I've learned that however tired I am, I can always manage a small piece of work, in fact, doing small chunks of work seems to be better for me.

And that reframe can end on the positive note:

Coach: That sounds great, learning how to learn is fundamental to doing well.

Reframing at first glance appears to be putting gloss on the dark side. In reality it helps the learner get a new perspective without belittling what they are doing, or tacitly agreeing with their view. It helps to get a new perspective, helping them change from thinking 'I can't do it' to 'yes, it may be tough at times, but I am getting somewhere'.

There are many reframes that we can and do use often quite conversationally. Here are a few examples. You will undoubtedly be able to think of more:

Examples

Outcome frame
- How else could this be?
- What do you want?
- What really matters to you in all this?

Backtrack frame
- To recap?
- What you are saying is ...?
- Can we retrace our steps ...?

Contrast frame
- How would it be if ...?
- Looking at this from another angle/in somebody else's shoes ...
- Could you sing this to a different tune?
- On the one hand I hear you saying this ..., but on the other hand I hear you also saying something else ...

'As if' frame:
- Suppose you did know ...?
- Try this on for size ...?
- If you were your hero how would it be, what would you do?
- Let's pretend ...
- If you had three wishes ...

Metaphor frame:
- What is this like?
- If this were a story what is the part that needs telling next?
- And what kind of X is that?
- And what happens next?

Voting

An advantage of a coaching approach is an increase in the number of choices available to the learner. The downside of this is that the learner now has to decide what they give priority to. Time is not unlimited. Learning when to say no, and when to say yes, are fundamental and learnable skills. Out of this can come a real sense of value, as well as the basic skill of better time keeping. How do they want to spend their time? How are they actually spending their time now? It can help if your coachee keeps a track of how they use their time for a week, to see how they are spending it. It might also help you, as their coach, to do it for your time too. Voting is partly about learning to say no, and partly about deciding how much time and energy to give to any part of your life.

Life is full of choices, and however much we would like to devote all our time to everything, we cannot. Voting helps the learner decide where they want to focus their energies; where, what and how they really want to be devoting their time to. It can help here to revisit the balance wheel, exploring again with the learner whether time spent on one segment is at the expense of another. Are they investing all their time in one segment of the balance wheel, voting for that at the expense of others? Are the choices our learner is making ones which support them? Is what they are voting for matching their values? Learners can leak energy in a variety of ways – they may concentrate on too much detail, or they may be stuck on thoughts of the past. When voting, the coach and learner explore what is really important to the learner – what is really important to them in terms of time, money and energy.

So you can vote with time – more time spent doing this rather than that. Or you can vote with money – choosing to spend it this way rather than that, choosing further learning or courses rather than expensive holidays. And the third way you can vote is with your energy – the things you think about, the mental environment you create, and the internal dialogues, or self-talk, you engage in.

Exercise

Think about your four or five top values (you can find out how to elicit these in Chapter 8 on values and beliefs). List them to one side of a sheet of paper. At the end of each day review how the day has been and record how you have voted for each of those values in terms of time, money and energy. Was the payoff worth it? Are there are other thoughts about the investment you made?

A simple chart as shown in Table 6.1 may help with this exercise.

From voting comes the idea of helping a learner plan. Tasks may seem to be big and unassailable when viewed as a whole, and learning how to chunk

Table 6.1   An example of a voting record chart

Value	Time	Money	Energy	Payoff

them down to a manageable size is helpful. For example the learner may say they really want to be able to work with people effectively, to which you, as coach, can ask: 'Could you do that today?', and the answer would probably be 'No' – 'Well, what could you do today?' – 'Well, I might be able to read about it'. 'And could you do that today?' 'No, I am not sure what books to use; I'd have to find out.' 'Could you do that today?' 'Yes, I could see what books there are in the library on the right sort of skills.' 'So today you will see what books there are in the library that could help you?' 'Yes, I will go and do that straight after this tutorial and see what I can find' – and you may even choose between you to hold them accountable to that.

So what seemed to be a big task has now been chunked down to something that is quite manageable and that the learner can go and do straight away. This can be very motivating.

Reference

1   Balint M (1957) *The Doctor, his Patient and the Illness*. International University Press, New York.

7

Meta-models and meta-programmes: why do people always . . .?

Going meta — what does that mean? The dictionary says it is something about being 'concerned with the concepts and results of a discipline'. Another way to imagine its meaning is to think of standing outside a teaching session you are having with your learner, looking at your interaction. There are several ways of looking at this. From your perspective, commonly called first position, you see the world from your point of view and experience the feelings that you have. If, on the other hand, you were to get into your learner's shoes, you would see the world from their viewpoint, understanding their feelings. This is often called second position. Third position is when you stand outside both you and your learner, looking at the interaction itself, getting a flavour of the whole process of teaching. This is the meta-position (Figure 7.1).

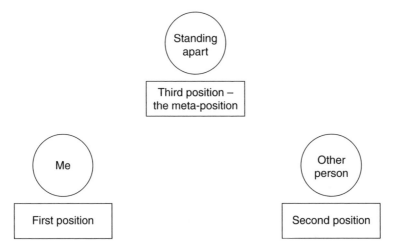

Figure 7.1 Perceptual positions.

Why does the learner never hear that nugget of information that you offer? Why does the learner always insist on examining the smallest detail of a case, when you know what is needed is a broad overview of the issues involved? To be able to do this, you need to go meta – either meta to the language which is being used (the meta-model) or meta to the way they are behaving (meta-programmes).

The meta-model

When listening to another person it is not possible to hear everything they say; we try to make meaning from it within our own understanding. This is really helpful to us or we would be cluttered with millions of pieces of redundant information. To help us retain useful information, our brains filter what we hear, trying to make sense of it, rejecting some things, adding others, and interpreting yet more.

There are three main ways we simplify:

- *deletion*: we leave information out
- *generalisation*: we make broad interpretations from limited evidence
- *distortion*: we make sense of what we hear by concentrating on some aspects, while ignoring others.

Too often as trainers we respond to these by mind-reading – we think we know what our learners are about to say and fill the answer in for them, either in words or in our heads. There are other ways of handling this, though, which match with the ideas of pacing the learner and working with their agenda.

Deletion

Your learner is telling you about a specific problem they had that morning. 'I find working with men so difficult – they don't listen to me. I don't know what to do,' they report. There are two deletions here. Who specifically does not listen to them? What specifically do they not know what to do about or to whom? Deletions suggest the learner is not completely clear in their own thoughts about what is going on, and by focusing in, you as coach will help them.

Another example would be where the learner is talking about finding it difficult to cope when people they are working with present written lists of the issues they need to consider. In exploring this she says 'yes but I want to make a good impression'. This could be taken at face value 'yes, we all do'. But in fact your learner has deleted some key information – who or what do they want to impress, and how do they want to impress them? Of greater interest would be to ask, 'How specifically do you want to impress that person?', with follow-up questions such as, 'And what would be the effect of that? On who?'

Generalisation

The next day you meet up with your learner to look at another problem issue. 'I thought I would discuss Mrs X with you, I always have problems with people who can't get to the point.' A response from you could be to challenge this generalisation. 'Always? You mean there is no time when you have no problems.' 'Well,' replies the learner, 'no, not always . . .', and then you can begin to tease out where there are similarities and differences.

Or perhaps your learner comes to say they have problems with another part of their training course and you are encouraging her to speak with the organiser. 'I can't speak to the organiser about this' she says. A common response to this might be, 'Why not?', and as so often happens with 'why' questions the dialogue may move into theoretical positions. Try asking instead, 'What would happen if you did?', or even, 'What stops you?', and notice how this opens new avenues and leads to options and choice. A major presupposition of the coaching approach is that the person you are working with, your learner, is resourceful. Hidden in them they have the potential to find a way through all their problems. Fundamental to this is the belief that your learner has choice and they, in the end, are responsible for the choices they make. Part of your role as coach is to help them see they have choices, explore those choices with them and then help them settle on the choice which they believe is best for them. And the more choice people have, the freer they are.

Distortion

On yet another day the learner asks to talk to you about a difficult problem she has had that morning. 'Mr Y was so difficult again – he makes me mad.' Here the learner has fallen into the cause–effect trap, that his behaviour *causes* her to feel mad. People, of course, cannot make others feel any way at all if they don't choose to, and one response might be to talk with your learner about this. An alternative response from you as a coaching trainer could challenge this link: 'How does his behaviour cause you to feel mad?' Or perhaps a counter example would be useful: 'Do you always feel mad when he behaves that way?', or you could even begin to unpack the strategy your learner uses: 'How specifically do you do *being mad*?'

Later in the discussion the same learner explains, 'I look too young to them, I know they think I haven't got the experience and don't know what I'm doing.' Some trainers may be tempted to agree with the problem or even reminisce about when they themselves were young, or perhaps they may even dismiss the issue out of hand: 'You don't look too young to me, or perhaps joke about it: 'Yes, even the police look young today.' It would be much more powerful to acknowledge the feeling and explore *that* with your learner: 'How do you know that?'; 'What lets you know?'

Key points about the meta-model

Deletion: what is the learner not saying?
Useful questions:

- Where? When? How? Who?
- Specifically, exactly.

Generalisation: are they using words like never or always?
Useful questions:

- All? Every? Never?
- What would happen if?
- What stops you?

Distortion: Are they making judgements or meanings which just aren't supported by evidence?
Useful questions:

- Who says?
- How do you know that?
- How does $x = y$?

Meta-programmes

These are largely unconscious patterns of behaviour, affecting what we notice, what we do, and how we sort and organise information. They determine the way we actually think. An analogy comes from computers. Many of us are familiar with the Windows environment, taking it for granted that it will, most of the time, run the programmes we want to use. Without Windows, your computer programmes would not run. Effectively it is the meta-programme within your computer. We too have operating systems that tell us how to see the world and how to interpret that world — these are called meta-programmes. In order to communicate effectively we need to observe a person carefully and listen to their language to understand how they are structuring their experience. It is important to know that there are no absolutes, that no one responds in exactly the same way to every situation. Few people operate at extremes either, but we do all develop preferred patterns of behaviour.

An example will help clarify this — your learner never seems to get to your tutorials on time. He is always immersed in what he is doing, lives life to the full, but has little regard for the clock. You, being punctual, and a good time-keeper find this more and more frustrating, making all sorts of suggestions to him, ranging from buying planners to going on a time management course. The truth is that you perceive time in different ways — your meta-programme is 'through-time'; you map time so that you can review and plan, by disassociating from the immediate moment so you can see how it relates to both past and future. People like you can often give a very accurate description of what happened in the past, and are quite likely to be able to say exactly what they will be doing a week from today. On the other hand your learner's meta-programme is 'in-time'. He lives in the moment, often being so

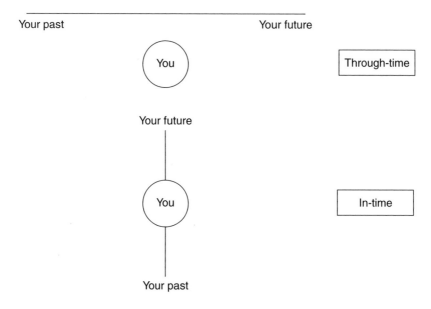

Figure 7.2   Two different time lines.

caught up in what is happening at any one time, that he completely loses track of time itself. People like him tend to have the past mapped behind them, with the future in front so they can literally not see where they are going. Time means little to them, it is not that they are rude or selfish, it is just a different way of seeing the world. Neither of the maps is wrong, both have merits, and both have disadvantages. Understanding where each other comes from can help avoid many misunderstandings (Figure 7.2).

Exercise

Try this, it is easy and fun! Practise on as many people as you can.

Ask the question 'point to the past' and then 'point to the future'.

Notice and be curious about the differences. Consider the impact of this on their perception of the world.

Now do it on yourself ...

Tip: Don't ask 'can you point to the past ...' The answer will be 'yes' or 'no', rather than an automatic reaction from their unconscious.

There are probably as many as 50 different meta-programmes, ranging from whether you prefer to see the big picture first or work with detail (chunk size), to whether you are an introvert or an extrovert. There seem to be about 10 that operate in most contexts, and of those, six or seven seem particularly relevant to coaching. It is useful to learn about the meta-programmes of your coachee, as it enables you to speak their language. It is also extremely useful to be aware of your dominant meta-programmes and to notice the similarities and differences between you and your learner.

Chunk size

This meta-programme is important for both learning and coaching. When people receive information in a size that matches their unconscious preferences they learn easily. If the information presented is too general or too detailed for them, they can easily lose interest. You can discover which of these meta-programmes runs in your coachee by recognising the patterns in their sentences.

Big chunk people like an overview first, talking in generalities, getting overwhelmed by detail. They will be at home with concepts and theories, liking summaries, and using simple sentences with little detail. You can appeal to big chunkers by beginning with big chunk statements like:

'What have you learnt so far?'

or

'That consultation was about feelings.'

Small chunk people like details, lists, and specific steps. They get bored with vagueness and generalities, drawing conclusions from small pieces of information or examples. They tend to speak in sequences, step by step with a lot of modifiers, adverbs and adjectives. You can appeal to these students by using lots of modifiers yourself and giving precise instructions in an ordered fashion, such as:

'This tutorial we are going to learn about models of communication. First we will cover theory, then verbal and non verbal communication, ending up with some practical tips which I am sure you will find very useful.'

Neither big nor small chunk is better than the other, and both are needed from time to time – it is how different people process the same information to make sense of it. What may happen is that the general person will follow specifics for a while, but will quickly get bored, whereas the specific person insists on giving more and more details to guarantee precision.

It is helpful to pace your coachee and match their language as much as possible. There are also times, however, when it can be extremely useful to challenge your coachee's meta-programmes. For example, your learner may have a small chunk meta-programme and be beginning to describe a particular situation: 'Well, you remember the day after the bank holiday, it was raining and traffic was dreadful. We were really busy, the new receptionist at work had just started and my appointments were running late. She really could not cope, she just sat there crying and I tried absolutely everything, and nothing worked, anyway I expect that is how it goes, so then I ...'. You as coach trainer could challenge this constructively by helping your learner see what really mattered in the story: 'What is really important about all this?' Or maybe you could help your learner chunk up to the real issue by asking them: 'What is all this an example of?' Both of these challenge the small chunk way of thinking and help the learner move towards being a big chunk thinker.

Contrast this with a big picture learner: 'Well, it was all about communication, just different wavelengths from the beginning. It got far too woolly and I could feel it all slipping away from the main point ...' Here you as trainer could help your learner develop a smaller chunk way of thinking by responding: 'Tell me exactly what the issue is? Give me a specific example of woolly? What would be an example of being on different wavelengths? What's the point here?'

In both these situations, challenging will move the learner forward to consider other perspectives, giving them choice in how they could generate new behaviours for themselves, and what they should be.

Options/procedures

Coachees with an options meta-programme are motivated by the possibility of doing things a different way. They love starting new projects, really enjoying the development and setup but may not be too bothered in finishing it. Committing themselves is hard as this will reduce their options. This meta-programme is closely related to the Myers-Briggs Type Indicator (MBTI) 'perceiver', who leaves it as late as possible to complete, just in case something new comes along.

A coachee with a procedures meta-programme, on the other hand, likes to follow set ways, there being a right way to do things. They tend to be completer-finishers, who are closely related to the MBTI 'judger'.[1]

You can see this meta-programme at work when a learner is preparing for an assessment. The procedures learner will look at the marking schedule and construct their work or project to fit this. This contrasts with the options learner who will be far more interested in novel ideas and different ways of looking at the problem. This learner can easily be bored by having to do something that fits in with someone else's framework. To them, creating a new framework is much more exciting.

Match/mismatch

Some coachees learn best by relating new information to what they already know; others prefer to look at how it is different from what they have experienced before.

Those with a sameness pattern (matchers) do not like change and find adapting difficult. They learn by noticing what is similar in situations, looking at what is common, and how things remain the same ... 'Isn't it interesting how the way Mrs Smith reacted to her problem was just the same as Mr Smith?'

Other people will emphasise how things are different, noticing what is missing. They understand by 'mismatching'. They tend to value new ways of doing things, quickly getting bored with things that remain static, and may even experiment to see what the new is like. They often notice mistakes their teacher or coach makes!

Few people are pure one or the other. Many first notice similarities then concentrate on difference, others the other way round, and yet others sort for sameness and difference about equally.

Coachees who agree with you, following your instructions diligently, may not be perfect students! They may rather just prefer to learn by matching. On the other hand, students who point out your inconsistencies and errors are actually making sense of the world by mismatching. Knowing this can transform the way you work with a 'difficult' coachee. So to engage a mismatcher, you need to explain how what they are learning is new and different. Contrast this with a matcher who needs to see how things are similar to what they already know, and how each idea builds on the last, helping them to see areas of continuity.

Convincer strategy

What specifically leads us to accept the believability of something? Until you are convinced, it is unlikely that you will take appropriate action. You and your coachee will generally have a preferred pattern for being convinced with two distinct parts – first, what sensory mode do you need to receive the information, and second how will you treat that information once you have it?

To elicit a coachee's convincer strategy, you might ask them how they know when to use a new way of doing something. Some will reply that they need to *see* some evidence, others will be convinced if they *hear* what someone such as a senior colleague says, yet others will be convinced by *reading* reports, and a fourth group will have to actually *practise* their new strategy and see its benefit before being convinced. This gives a clue to the convincer channel, whether it is see, hear, read or do.

On top of this, once information has been gathered, the coachee will need to use it in some way before they are really convinced about it. For some it is just automatic, one example is enough. For others, they need to have the data a certain number of times to be convinced. Some people are never really convinced – I'll judge each case on its merits. Then the final group need to gather information over a period of time to be convinced – I'll use this new strategy for a year before it becomes one of my habits.

This clearly has relevance to learning, because as coach you need to know how best to help your coachee get the information they need to practise.

Toward/away from

What will trigger your coachee to action? Do they respond best to the carrot or the stick? The two patterns in this category describe either moving toward a goal, or away from a problem.

'Toward' coachees are focused on their goal, being motivated to achieve, and getting excited and energised by these goals. They tend to talk about what they will gain. This group may be more motivated by carrots. They will often minimise negative consequences, and will have difficulty identifying what to avoid. These coachees can appear very self-motivating, but it is important to be aware that they may ignore potential problems.

'Away from' coachees are motivated by a problem to be solved, or when there is something to move away from. They tend to talk about situations to be avoided. They learn because they find a gap in their knowledge, and so move away from this by acquiring new knowledge or skills. This group may be more motivated by sticks.

It can be helpful to ask them what they don't want, for example don't ask them, 'What would you like to do in the next conversation you have with Mr Jones, a person I know you find particularly difficult?'; instead you could try asking, 'What don't you want to happen ...?'

It is important to know that many people can at first appear to have a toward meta-programme. On closer questioning and listening, however, it can quickly become clear that they have a primary motivation of 'moving away from', followed by 'moving towards'.

Internal/external frame of reference

This meta-programme is very important when giving feedback to your coachee. An internally referenced coachee just knows when they have done a good job; if you ask them how they know when they have done a good job they typically reply something like 'it feels like it's gone well', or 'I just know'. An externally referenced coachee on the other hand will need to be told they are doing well, they enjoy feedback, in fact need it. So an externally referenced coachee must have feedback from you as coach for them to be able to evaluate their progress. If you ask a strongly external individual how they think they are doing they will probably respond, 'Well ... how do *you* think I'm doing?' For example, this coachee will respond to examples and facts such as, 'One of my previous learners found this very useful and those that couldn't found it harder to prepare for exams.'

An internally referenced person who is asked how they think they are doing is likely to give a direct answer. They know and are confident in that knowing. Strongly internally referenced students can actually resent feedback, especially if it contradicts their own opinion. They are motivated by their own evaluation of how much progress they have made, and may think, 'Who are you to tell me?' Giving feedback to such a coachee needs to be tackled with care, directing attention to their focus of how they are doing. It might be appropriate to word the feedback something like: 'I'd like to hear how you think you are doing, so we can talk about your progress', or 'I know I can't convince you to go on this course of study as you are the only one who knows the benefits of going' – though you may want to rephrase this for an away from learner to 'how you will miss out if you don't go'.

So how do you find out which is your coachee's preferred meta-programme here? One way to find out is to ask them: 'If you think you have just had a really good conversation with someone, yet you overhear that person later telling a friend how bad it had been, what do you straight away think?' If they reply, 'What do they know, they weren't there' or 'Well I thought it was OK' you can be pretty sure your coachee is internally referenced. If they replied, 'I'd feel terrible' then they are externally referenced.

Of course, nobody is totally externally or internally referenced. However, when somebody has a preference you can very quickly lose respect and rapport by not communicating with them in their preferred style.

Exercise

To some this may all sound very straightforward and obvious. To others it is very confusing. In reality it can be tricky picking up these verbal and non-verbal cues and responding to them in an appropriate way. It takes a lot of practice.

Select one meta-programme that you want to practise picking up. For a whole week listen to people you come across, members of your family, friends, colleagues, your learner, clients, whoever. Practise listening for the cues. Experiment with different ways of responding and feel the results. Ask for feedback. See if you are right in what you are thinking. Get a feeling for what works and what doesn't work. Hear what people say.

How do you confront your coachee?

Confront is a strong word. How did you feel when you read it? We debated for some time whether this was a good word to use, and felt that it conveyed the fact that telling your coachee something which will be difficult to hear can feel confrontational to many, yet to others it can seem easy. As you may imagine, it all depends on your meta-programmes! The essence is to consider how best to bring things up so that the coachee really does hear what you want them to hear.

First, not to confront your coachee is devaluing them – if you know an area where they can change it is not ethical to ignore it.

Second, it is important to establish whether you have to work at the identity, values, capability or behaviour level. This concept is explored elsewhere under the heading 'Logical levels' (p. 46).

Third, it is always important to remember that it is your responsibility as the trainer or coach to ensure that the message you want your learner to hear is given in such a way that they do hear it. In the end, the meaning of your communication is the response that you get from your learner. People respond to what they think you mean – this may or may not be an accurate interpretation of what you intended to mean. You need to be constantly aware of how your learner is responding to what you are saying, adjusting what you are saying accordingly, rather than just assuming that they will have understood what you meant them to understand. It's worth also considering what resources you are going to need to help you with this.

Fourth, it is helpful to disassociate from the message by using the past tense, by not using the word 'you', by gesturing away from your coachee, and by avoiding generalisations. Remember that traditionally it is the messenger who gets hurt by delivering bad news – and remember for your learner when you confront them it is bad news. You can help avoid this by displacing yourself from the message, by, for example, writing the message down on a piece of paper and pointing to that while looking away from your learner. A change of voice tone and posture can also help. Follow the message by a pause, and then as you look back to your learner your voice tone and tempo can rise as you explore with your learner what they could do differently. This way the learner disassociates from the bad news, immediately followed by re-associating into looking at appropriate remedies.

These moves can be encapsulated by the notion of the feedback sandwich. Start with a positive statement about the person – at the identity level. Move to looking at the behaviour which needs to change, remembering to keep it at the behaviour level. Finish the sandwich by exploring with your coachee what they need to do to make appropriate changes; this is working now at the capability level, and ends the session on a positive note.

You can help all this by thinking about your learner's values for improving (which you will have explored at their intake session and subsequently) and aligning what you say with these values. It is helpful to believe that all actions have a positive intention, as far as the person exhibiting the behaviour is concerned, whatever the outcome. This neither means that the behaviour is the best possible choice nor that the behaviour will have positive benefits for anyone else other than the learner. One solution to inappropriate behaviour is to find a way of satisfying the intention behind it by more acceptable means. Working with your learner's positive intentions in this way can also give focus and direction to what they do, and is more likely to be successful.

A summary of useful meta-programmes and how to elicit them

- Time:
  - *In-time (i.e. time stored from front, present and future, to back, past)*: see events as unrelated, tend to associate into memories, often late, get caught up in the here and now, tend to be more interested in starting rather than finishing projects, make quick decisions
  - *Through-time (i.e. time stored left to right in front of them)*: see events as related, time can seem long, continuous, no interruptions, slow to decide, tend to be on time, collapse memories into one common gestalt, so find it hard to recall specifics, need to complete and close
- Chunk size:
  - *Big picture*: essentially, most important, main idea; usually use short simple sentences.
  - *Small picture*: precisely, specifically, for example, lots of adjectives and adverbs; if they are interrupted will often go back to the beginning.
- Options/procedures:
  - *Options*: many ways to skin a cat, reluctant to start in case a better idea comes along, create outlines and procedures but hate following them.
  - *Procedures*: want to know the right way to do things, anxious about change or not following every step.
- Match/mismatch:
  - *Match*: same, just like, similar to, in common, maintain.
  - *Mismatch*: 'night and day', different, unique, radical, new.
- Toward/away from:
  - *Toward*: want, gain, have, accomplish, like, include people and things.
  - *Away from*: don't want, avoids, anticipate problems, exclude things and people.
- Internal/external frame of reference:
  - *Internal*: it feels right, I just know, resist decisions made for them by others.
  - *External*: someone has to tell me, the facts speak for themselves, they will say thank you, that's the way it is.

Reference

1   Bayne R (2004) *Psychological Types at Work: An MBTI Perspective*. Thomson Learning, London.

8

Beliefs and values

'Aha, I've got you now,' grins the coachee triumphantly, 'it's what I believe and you can't change beliefs!'
'Have you ever believed in Father Christmas or the tooth fairy?' responds the coach.

Henry Ford is reputed to have said, 'Whether you think you can or whether you think you can't, you are probably right'. By saying that, he confirmed the common wisdom that if a person believes they can do something they will, and if they believe something is impossible no amount of effort will convince them to accomplish it. Rosenthal in 1985 showed that students whose teachers thought they were high performers performed better than those whose teachers did not believe in them.[1]

Beliefs colour our world. They are powerful determinants of our behaviour and our capabilities. When we believe something to be true, about ourselves or about the world, it becomes our reality. We organise and frame our experiences in ways that will tend to confirm what we believe. Education is a perfect example of the power of beliefs on performance. Our beliefs are often formed very early on in life. As coaches we hear these beliefs expressed by adult learners and see the impact they have on the process of learning. The beliefs range from 'I can do anything', to 'I am useless at learning'; from 'Well, it's worth taking a risk and getting it wrong' to 'I mustn't submit anything that is less than perfect'; from 'Learning is fun' to 'Learning is frightening' or 'Learning is boring'. Take a moment to ask yourself, 'What do I believe about education and learning?' And now consider how your life would have been different if you had believed something different about education.

Beliefs are fundamental to how we integrate new information and to how we make decisions. They determine how we code our memories and how we live the story of our lives. There is a living tapestry of examples of this: think of the woman who believes that she is a victim to all that life throws at her, who then develops breast cancer ... how will she tell her story? Think of the man who believes that he must remain in control at all times ... how will he react when he loses his job? Think of the learner who believes that there is always a right answer ... how will she frame the experience of uncertainty in her education? People tell us their stories, and if we listen carefully we can hear the beliefs that bind the book of their life together. We can see the frames that they put around the illustrations. If we step out and see the movie and sound track of our own experiences, we will start to notice how our own beliefs have impacted on us.

People behave as if their beliefs are true and fixed. Yet the reality is that beliefs get updated and changed as we go through life. The process of belief change is generally subtle and often unconscious. It is only when we reflect and look back to where we have been and how we used to behave, that we may notice the change. Father Christmas and tooth fairies are obvious examples, but there are many others. How have your beliefs about teachers changed? How about exams and assessment? How has what you believe about love and money determined what you have done so far in life? Our beliefs have a profound effect on our life, yet we rarely acknowledge them let alone explore or challenge them.

The role of the coach is to draw on the learner's own strengths and resources so they can develop in the way that they choose. These strengths and resources exist at more than just the behavioural and capability level. Lasting change and continuing personal development occurs when we are congruent at the highest levels – congruent with our beliefs, values and identity. It occurs when we discover our unconscious competencies and overcome internal resistance and limiting beliefs. The coach can work with a learner's beliefs by identifying them, honouring them and exploring them respectfully to establish a hierarchy that is true for the coachee. By raising beliefs to conscious awareness, the mind starts to create new links and becomes aware of alternatives and choice. The coach who works purely at the behavioural or capability level will not open the doors of lasting change and continued growth to the coachee. Let me give you an example of this before we look at the facts and 'how to' of working with beliefs.

Example

Consider a learner who, after any success, instantly focuses on the next hurdle. 'Yes, I know I just handled that well, but that was because we had discussed it first. What I really want to do is to be naturally assertive without planning.' The effect of this sort of thinking is twofold. First it wipes out the benefit of praise or celebration, and negates the learning in that experience, and second it creates a natural anti-success strategy where nothing is ever good enough. The beliefs driving this thinking could be many, and the coach cannot even guess or assume what these may be. In this example, the coach merely reflected back to the coachee their repeated pattern of behaviour and what she saw to be the consequences. 'So, I'm just curious about what might be driving this,' the coach asks. 'Well … I've always got to do my best,' replies the coachee, 'and this isn't my best.' Now the conversation flows along the lines of what is best, for whom, when, and whether there is something more important than doing your best.

Working with beliefs

To work with beliefs, we have to understand something about what they are and how they are expressed. Here are some facts about beliefs:

- Beliefs are generalisations that we hold to be true.
- They relate to causation, meaning and boundaries around our identity, our behaviour, our skills and the world around us.
- Beliefs are very powerful.
- Beliefs provide the motivation and permission that supports or inhibits particular behaviour.
- Beliefs relate to the question 'why?'
- Beliefs are notoriously difficult to change through logic and rational thought.
- Our most influential beliefs are often outside conscious awareness.
- Beliefs are like onions, held together in layers.
- Beliefs change.

There is an old story that beautifully demonstrates many of these facts. A patient being treated by a psychiatrist claims that he is a corpse and so doesn't have to eat or take care of himself. The psychiatrist spends hours presenting the rational arguments as to why the patient is not a corpse. Finally he asks if corpses bleed. The patient looks at him as if he is stupid, 'Of course they don't bleed, all their body functions have stopped.' They agree to carry out an experiment where the psychiatrist will prick the patient with a needle to see if he bleeds. Sure enough the patient bleeds, and with a look of amazement he gasps, 'I'll be darned … corpses *do* bleed.'

The origin and language of beliefs

We acquire our beliefs through myriad sources, our families, society, experience, religion, education. At different times of our lives our beliefs may be challenged, and then we get to question our beliefs. If we have someone around us to prompt those questions we are more likely to pay attention and centre ourselves in the core of what is important to us, rather than being driven by beliefs that do not belong to us any more. This is the role of the coach. The coach assumes that all our beliefs, even our limiting beliefs, fulfil, or have in the past fulfilled, a useful purpose. The useful purpose is often around issues such as protection, establishing boundaries of right and wrong, or around personal power and control. These are profound purposes, and so fundamental that we rarely stop and consider whether a particular belief is actually serving that purpose in the best way, let alone whether another belief would serve us better.

So inherent are beliefs in our nature, and so tied up with our personal sense of identity that they are rarely discussed openly. So, beliefs are inferred through our behaviour and through our language. Words such as *should/ shouldn't, can/can't, ought, always, never, good, right*, give clues to an underlying generalisation or belief. Statements such as *'this just isn't me, I don't know what it's all about'*, or *'it doesn't make sense but . . .', 'it sounds crazy but . . . , I just can't'!*, suggest an impasse relating to a belief.

As coach, the significance is to be aware of this in your learner. The art is to gently probe while acknowledging the deep intention of beliefs and respecting the identity of the learner.

Questions you may ask include:

- What is this all about?
- What is the bottom line here?
- Where is this coming from?
- What stops you?
- Is that what you really believe?
- Does this belief really belong to you? Whose belief is it?
- How does it help you now to believe this?
- What would happen if . . .?
- What do you want to believe instead?
- How would it be if you did believe that?

The coach raises the belief, or even the notion of an underlying belief, to conscious awareness. There is no question of right or wrong. There is no rational explanation or counter explanation to be sought. There is only the opening of a window to a view of wondering and questioning. It is for the coachee to choose whether to draw the curtains or not.

Some of these questions assume that changing beliefs is possible. Your learner may not agree: 'Well, of course I'd like to believe that learning is easy, but that can't just happen.' A gentle introduction and a good pacing exercise for someone with this mind set is to ask them to consider the following exercise:

Exercise

Beliefs through time (adapted from Ian McDermott and Jan Elfline)[2]

Identify what you thought about each of these words when you were at each of the ages listed. Notice how they have changed. If you haven't reached one of the ages listed here, guess what you might think when you reach that age. Fill in the chart (Table 8.1).

Table 8.1 Beliefs changing with time

	Child	15	25	35	45	55	65	75
Religion								
Sex								
Money								
Success								
40-year-olds								
Intelligence								
Love								
Work								
Learning								
Appearance								

This is a fun exercise to share with a learner. You can change the rows to suit your purpose and play with what you might believe when you are 100 years old. More profoundly this exercise starts to question the assumption that beliefs can't change and leads naturally into questions such as:

- What could you believe?
- What will you always believe?

- What might you like to believe?
- What would you need?
- So what do you believe about ...?

Limiting beliefs

Beliefs can serve us very well. They can also hold us back. We all have beliefs which limit us in some way. That is to say, they do not serve us in the best way to help us achieve what we claim we want. These limiting beliefs are especially common around education. They commonly originate in the dim and distant past, and are a result of formative, usually negative, experiences. These experiences remain locked within the perspective of the younger, less understanding self. They become transformed into beliefs which encourage self-perpetuating behaviour and self-perpetuating interpretation of associated experiences. Phrases such as 'my teacher always said I was hopeless at maths', and 'I dreaded my parents seeing my results', are all too common. Just mention the word assessment, and many adults break into a cold sweat at the thought of judgement and failure. The impact on our learning and development and on our physical and mental wellbeing is enormous.

Limiting beliefs commonly centre around three broad themes: hopelessness, helplessness and worthlessness.

- *Hopelessness*: the belief that the desired outcome is not achievable regardless of your abilities. 'That will never happen, no matter what'; 'I will never be well again.'
- *Helplessness*: the belief that the desired outcome is possible but you are not capable of achieving it. 'Yes, I know it can be done but not by me.'
- *Worthlessness*: the belief that you do not deserve the desired goal because of something you are or have (not) done. 'I don't deserve that'; 'Happiness is for others not for me.'

Here are some common limiting beliefs around learning:

- I'm not good enough.
- No matter how hard I try, I'll never be able to do that.
- Learning is boring.
- Learning is hard work.
- I've got a useless memory.
- I'm not creative.
- I was rubbish at school.

- I am a failure.
- I'm too old to learn anything new.
- They'll think I'm no good/stupid.
- It's no good unless it's perfect.
- It's scary to try new things.

All of these have a positive intention which in some way serves the learner. Around each of these there are also some assumptions and unanswered 'how to' questions. In order to challenge the limiting belief the coach will ask questions such as:

- How can you try something new and stay safe?
- How can you be enough?
- Tell me about something you remember really well. And how do you do that? (self-modelling).
- How would it be if you believed that you could learn new things?
- How could you make learning easy and fun?
- How do you know that you were rubbish at school? What do you really believe?
- How do want to see/think of yourself? And how is it when you think of yourself in this new way?
- How do know what is perfect?
- How can you do 'not perfect'?

These questions percolate through consciousness to the unconscious level, to question assumptions. Dropping a little pebble creates the ripples of possibility of other ways of being. Apparently casual, small questions can have a tremendous impact that you as coach may or may not be around to see.

Beliefs and motivation

We have already looked at how we can help learners to define what they want and to create well-formed outcomes ('What do you want' in Chapter 4). That is an incredible first step to planning and implementing behavioural change. This process of change is supported by a belief system about how we reach our outcomes. As with all beliefs, they are often out of conscious thought and need prompting to undergo conscious examination. An evaluation of these beliefs is especially worthwhile where there appears to be a discrepancy between what people say they want, and their motivation or progress.

The belief issues about change and achieving our outcomes centre around five key areas. These are based on work by Robert Dilts who has published extensively on transforming belief.[3] They are best summarised as statements:

1 The outcome is desirable and worthwhile.
2 It is possible for me to achieve this outcome.
3 What I have to do in order to achieve this is appropriate and fits with my sense of self.
4 I have the skills and capabilities to achieve this.
5 I am responsible for achieving this.
6 I deserve this.

Let us put this into context by looking at an example of a learner who wants to develop their communication skills:

1 *Desirability*: all things being equal most people would want this. But life is not equal, we have hierarchies of wants. The learner may say, 'Well, I need to be more confident in my knowledge base first' or perhaps 'I have a family crisis right now that needs my energy'
2 *Achievability*: from here may emerge many beliefs. Some that we have heard include: 'Well, fundamentally you can't change who you are', or 'I might learn a few tricks but will it be me — they'll see through it and see me for what I am', 'But if I feel uncertain and anxious there's nothing I can do to hide that'
3 *Appropriate behaviour*: the learner may have a deep desire to learn new skills and believe that it is achievable, but have doubt about the process of getting there. For example a video may have other consequences that are apparently too big to confront, or a course may seem appropriate but the impact on family life at that time is too big a price to pay
4 *Capabilities*: the learner may be very positive about the first three but have low confidence in their own abilities. For example 'I have just gone through a divorce despite trying to make it work . . . if I can't do it for the most important part of my life, how can I do it for work', or 'I'm just not focused enough', or 'I feel too detached'
5 *Responsibility and self-worth*: a learner may believe that, 'It is up to the experts to teach me this; it is not my responsibility to learn it.' Learners may also doubt whether they deserve to succeed and be good. If a learner doesn't believe that they deserve to reach an outcome and they are not responsible for it, then, whatever else they believe, they will not get there. This then will be the first area of exploration.

In practical terms it is useful to explore and record these areas with your learner in a rating scale exercise. This gives an immediate visual profile of potential blocks in motivation or confidence. Get them to write down an outcome about themselves that they want:

Exercise

Belief rating scale

Outcome: . . . .

Please rate your degree of belief and confidence in the outcome in relation to each of the following statements by ringing around a number; 1 is the lowest (I don't believe this, no way) and 5 the highest (I believe this absolutely), with 3 being the answer 'maybe'.

The outcome is desirable and worth it for me
1   2   3   4   5

I can achieve this outcome
1   2   3   4   5

What I have to do is appropriate and fits with who I am
1   2   3   4   5

I have the capabilties to achieve this outcome
1   2   3   4   5

I have the responsibility for doing this
1   2   3   4   5

I deserve this
1   2   3   4   5

Adapted from Robert Dilts[2]

Having assessed the degree of confidence, the coach can then explore areas of doubt with the learner. The key assumption for the coach here is that we can change our beliefs to serve us better. Questions to ask include:

- What else would you need in order to be more confident?
- What would happen if you brought more strength/humour/compassion to that belief?
- What is true here?
- Are you beginning to question this belief?
- Are you open to the possibility of a different way of thinking?
- What belief would serve you better?
- How would it be to believe that?

Beliefs of the coach

As a coach to your learner you are enabling both of you to discover more about what makes them tick. What drives them forward? What holds them back? What is important? What do they want? How do they see their world? Now, what about you ... what do you believe about your role? We have talked previously of the importance of setting intention and of being curious and non-judgemental. To be genuine and congruent in this you need a set of beliefs to support you.

In the research mentioned at the beginning of this chapter, Rosenthal randomly divided a group of children of average intelligence into two even groups.[1] One of the groups was assigned a teacher who was told that the children were 'gifted'. The other group was given to a teacher who was told that her pupils were 'slow learners'. A year later the two groups were retested on the same intelligence measure. Not surprisingly, most of the group labelled gifted scored higher than previously, while most of the 'slow learners' scored lower. The teachers' beliefs about the students affected their ability to learn.

Exercise

Take some quiet and time when you won't be distracted to think about what you believe about yourself as a teacher/coach. Ask yourself these questions and write down the answers:

- How do I think of myself as a teacher/coach?
- What do I believe is my role?
- What is most important to me in this role?
- What are my strengths?
- What should my relationship with my learners be?
- What is my relationship with learners?
- What do I believe about my learners?
- What responsibility do I have to them?
- What responsibility do they have to me?

And now think of yourself as a learner, still growing and still developing new skills in coaching:

- How am I as a learner?
- What do I think of my teachers?
- What do I want to get better at?
- Where am I playing helpless or being passive?

- Which of my teachers are my role models? Who do I want to emulate?
- What is the stretch for me as a teacher/coach?
- Who do I want to be?
- What do I want to believe about me as a coach?

By writing down the answers you commit and focus. This in itself could be the most powerful piece of self-development work that you do as a coach for yourself. It will undoubtedly affect how you are as a coach and how your learner gains from you.

Values

Values and beliefs are intimately connected. Values are notions that we hold to be important and worthwhile. A value may be supported by a number of different beliefs. For example the value of freedom may be supported by a belief such as 'I believe it is OK to break rules that I don't agree with', or by 'I believe that thoughts are what cage people in'. It is common nowadays to hear people talk about their values. It is important as a coach to be aware of what values are and what they are not. It is important to recognise the significance of values in how people do what they do.

Let us start with what values are not – they are *not* morals. There is no sense of right and wrong, of positive or negative. Values are not about moral behaviour, though someone may have the value honesty, and that may or may not drive their own ethical behaviour. Similarly values are not inherently virtuous; they are intrinsic to us and not consciously chosen. What is important is our ability to live our values fully in our lives.

Values are about who we are, not who we would like to be. When we honour our values there is a sense of congruency and integrity. We feel 'right' inside and we have a sense of fulfilment. An individual's hierarchy of values determines the essence of who they are. When we do not live out our values, there is discord inside us. We are able to absorb a huge amount of dissonance; however there comes a point where the price we pay is too much in terms of our mental, emotional and physical wellbeing. We then live a life of tolerating rather than of happiness and fulfilment.

Values are like filters of worth through which we sort experience and create and judge our own behaviour. Values serve as compasses in our decision making. They can be difficult to name, and we are often shy about articulating powerful words such as peace or freedom which we are aware can mean different things to different people. In order to get the meaning we can group values, for example love/compassion/helping others are different from love/spirituality/happiness. Because values are often intangible it is important that we look for an individual's own definition, and not one from a dictionary. Other examples of values are independence, flexibility, intimacy, humour, creativity. (See Box 8.1 at the end of the chapter for a list of values.) Money in itself is not a value, but it may give you values such as security, fun, or service to others. Travelling is not a value, but it may support important values such as freedom, adventure, learning or spirituality.

Although values can be intangible they are not invisible. You can walk into a room of strangers and get a sense of what people value by the way they relate to each other or by what they are wearing. When you work or live with someone you get to know about things that are really important to them, such as timekeeping or flexibility, or being true to their word. The degree to which we live our values and demonstrate them in day-to-day behaviour varies. For some the value of honesty is absolute, to the extent that they feel it necessary to be brutally honest to friends about everything. For others, the boundary with values of kindness and tolerance blurs the edges, and their response may be more tempered. Our hierarchy of values affects how we behave in different situations. For example, if financial security is a high value we may tolerate hypocrisy in a job, yet at home, where trust is a key value, we may become very angry at even a hint of dishonesty. Communication with others is helped if we can understand and express what, in a given situation, is important to us. In a learning environment, a coach elicits and makes overt the values that drive different behaviour and motivation for the learner. These values will be unique to each individual. Recognising and acknowledging their values gives the learner clarity and aids decision making.

Eliciting values

Informal/conversational

The importance of values in coaching is that we all have a hierarchy of values which are supported by different beliefs. Values affect decision making in terms of the 'rightness' of choices. When learning is supported by honouring our values, it is easier, more fun and more directed. The learner also feels congruent. There are times however when values may clash or are not being honoured. This will manifest itself in terms of an apparent lack of motivation or a learner just not feeling 'right'. So it is valuable for the coach to notice times of choice and decision making, and to elicit the underlying values. A clue that there may be a clash of values is when you detect signs of incongruence in your learner. By incongruence we mean a sense of a person saying one thing but thinking or meaning another, a sense that something is being held back, or that they are not fully aligned emotionally and intellectually. Imagine watching your 16-year-old son thanking Aunt Mildred for the pink crochet napkin holder she has made him. There is likely to be incongruence. Now imagine him thanking his granddad for the scooter that will enable him to get to college on his own − here there will be congruence. It is also important for us as coaches to recognise signs of congruence in ourselves, that sense of certainty, of standing tall and going fully with a decision, as opposed to the signs of incongruence when we are more likely to procrastinate and offer 'yes but' excuses.

Questions that will help you and your learner in these situations are:

- What is important to you here?
- What is most important?
- What would mean that you could absolutely not do this?
- Which values will you be honouring when you do this?
- How will doing this serve you?
- What is the tension here?

In a coaching environment the aim is to draw learning from past experiences. Carrying this learning forward in terms of understanding the values behind it is more likely to result in deeper, longer-lasting change in behaviour. We can change behaviour temporarily but if we do not really hold it to be important we are likely to slip back to our old patterns. Then we hear ourselves saying things like 'oh yes I keep doing that', or 'I don't know why I just can't remember to do that'. When we are congruent we don't have to actively 'remember' anything − life is easier.

Questions that generate this sort of thinking include:

- What was important there that you held on to?
- What values were violated?
- What felt right? What grated with you?
- What were the consequences?
- What is the learning?
- What will you do next time?

Clarifying values in this way allows learners to acknowledge the significance of values in terms of strategies that they use. Done in a supportive way it also promotes a questioning curiosity, and the learner will start to recognise for themself situations where values are an issue. The learner starts to look at situations in terms of what is the bottom line, what I am prepared to do and what I am not. Decisions become more certain and are more likely to be carried through.

Structured approach

In apprenticeship models of learning, and in formal coaching there is a valuable place for a structured elicitation of values. This has two purposes — it serves as a 'getting to know you' exercise (as described in Chapter 3 on designing the alliance) that can then be revisited and refined later in training, and it also helps to create a focus and a way of working together.

We can witness values through behaviour, yet the process of unpicking and naming our own values can be difficult. We find that people either intellectualise and agonise over precise meaning and labels, or that they fantasise about which values would be 'good'. The trick here is to get people to look at their day-to-day lives, warts and all, in order to uncover the values that are informing daily actions and interactions. There is a list of values in Box 8.1 at the end of the chapter — we recommend using this as a prompt and illustration of some possible values. Used alone, a list is likely to generate analytical thought and debate. A skilled coach will elicit values from a 'heart' rather than 'head' perspective by taking clients into real-life situations. As you do this, remember that it is often easier to list a string of related values in order to avoid getting lost in debate over meaning; fun means different things to different people — as long as the learner knows what it means then that's fine.

Setting the scene

Here is the sort of language we use when describing values before taking a learner into more specific areas:

> Your values help you make choices about what you commit to in your life. They are so much part of you that you are hardly aware of them. If you commit time and energy to something that violates or neglects one of your core values, you will start feeling resentful or frustrated or perhaps just get that niggling feeling that something is not quite right. Not honouring values when you make choices about activities or relationships will give you a sense that something is not quite right with your life. Values here means the qualities that make you who you are, the real core of what makes you you. Without these things you would not be you. There isn't a right answer to any of these questions, you may find a string of words or a sentence or paragraph works better for you.

Discovering the values

To elicit values we look at four different areas of life. Depending on the person each area may resonate more or less. The four areas are:

- peak experiences
- 'drive you crazy' scenarios
- hidden values
- 'must haves'.

We like to explore these areas using an 'APC' approach.

Peak experiences

Ask: When has life been rich, full and exhilarating? It may be momentary, or maybe it lasted longer, a week, a month or perhaps even longer. What was important about the experience?

Probe: Who was there? What was going on? What was important to you?

Clarify: Get specific on detail. You might ask questions such as: 'What does achievement mean to you?', 'Sounds like there was something about being part of a team, is that right?', 'What is it?'

'Drive you crazy' scenarios

Ask: Think of a time when you have been sad or cross or frustrated. What drives you crazy or makes you angry or frustrated? If you think about one of those things, which of your values is being violated? What is that you can't live with and still be true to yourself?

Probe: A recurrent theme here seems to be around hypocrisy. If we turn this around to look for the value it could be around honesty or integrity, what rings true for you?

Clarify: Again, get specific – 'The frustration around moving goal posts is that about finishing a job or is it about finding a purpose?'

Hidden values

Ask: What is so much a part of you that you haven't even thought about it. You may find answers to this pop in your mind when you least expect them to. It's worth keeping a note book or jotter handy to capture such elusive thoughts!

Probe: What do others say about you? When you get teased about always going on about something, what is it? Examples include 'always late' or 'no idea of time' or 'so controlling'.

Clarify: Focus on the positives behind these values asking: 'What is this all about', 'What value drives this?'

'Must haves'

Ask: What is important to you? What do you care about? What do you want in your life? What can you not live without?

Probe: What values must you absolutely honour otherwise you wouldn't be you (that is a very tough question – think about it for yourself).

Clarify: And what does having this give you day to day?

Ranking values

So you can make best use of all the information you have elicited, it is important to now categorise your values. We ask the learner to pick their top 10 values, and then to rank the top three or four.

Living values score

To illuminate the learning still further the learner is now asked to score each value out of 10 according to how well they are being honoured in life, right now. The usual scale is; 1 is low (not being honoured at all), and 10 is high (fully honoured).

So you may end up with a list like this;

- peace 5/10
- freedom 2/10
- participation 8/10
- success 7/10
- humour 8/10

Seeing this alone is a powerful experience – try it for yourself. It also opens the door to further exploration and gentle challenge as different circumstances emerge. It enables an extra and powerful currency that can be used consciously and overtly in personal and professional development.

Decision making with values

As we have discussed, the hierarchy of values can change in different situations. For example, the value of fun may be very high in leisure but less high at work. When making a choice it is helpful to compare and contrast the ranking of values. Having elicited the top four values A, B, C and D, we then ask, 'If you could choose between a situation that gives you A and the one that gives you B, which would you go for?' By doing this for the each of the values, a hierarchy emerges which is valuable and often quite surprising. This is a good exercise to use when people are stuck between choices and say things like 'well I'm not sure' or 'on the one hand ... but on the other ...' or 'I just can't work this out, I'll toss a coin'. Eliciting the hierarchy of values in this way gives voice to those feelings and concepts, and enables the learner to decide what is more or less important in a given context.

Example

John is trying to choose a degree programme. Together you have elicited the top four values that are important to him. They are: money, flexibility, challenge and working face to face with people.

The conversation could go like this:

Coach: So we know what is important to you and what you want in a course. Let's imagine that course X is considerably cheaper and course Y would give greater flexibility. Which one attracts you?
John: Y – the one with flexibility.
Coach: Now imagine course X gives you flexibility and course Y provides the greater intellectual challenge. Which would you prefer?
John: Still flexibility.
Coach: Course X gives you flexibility, and course Y allows you to learn face to face. Which appeals now?
John: I really want flexibility at the moment.
Coach: OK, so we know that at the moment in terms of choosing a course, flexibility is most important for you.

Now, in the same way, you go on to compare the other values with each other and a hierarchy will emerge which could be:

1   flexibility
2   working face to face
3   challenge
4   money.

John can now look at the courses available; he may choose one or he may decide to delay until there is another opportunity which better fits his criteria. Whatever he decides, he will be clear about how he made his decision, and he will be congruent and settled within himself.

You may choose to do this exercise for yourself over any choice in life – it's particularly helpful when a team is having problems deciding what option to choose, as our choices are so often governed by our values, and disagreements often happen when core values clash. It's also very useful when we take major decisions in life, like which house to buy!

Working with values is one of the most challenging areas in coaching. It can also be the most rewarding. It raises a coaching conversation from chat to dealing with deep issues things that really matter to people.

Box 8.1 gives some suggestions to prompt you about values should you need it.

Box 8.1   Values list

Accuracy	Acknowledgement	Adventure
Authenticity	Awareness	Beauty
Being professional	Challenge	Choice
Collaboration	Communication	Community
Compassion	Contribution	Creativity
Discovery	Elegance	Empathy
Empowerment	Environment	Equality
Excellence	Fairness	Fitness
Flexibility	Focus	Free spirit
Freedom to choose	Friendship	Honesty
Humour	Independence	Integrity
Joy	Justice	Leadership
Learning	Lightness	Love
Merit	Nurturing	Optimism
Orderliness	Patience	Personal growth
Personal power	Productivity	Reliability
Respect	Responsibility	Risk taking
Romance	Service	Spirituality
Success	To be known	Trust
Truth	Vitality	Zest

Reference

1   Rosenthal R (1985) From unconscious experimenter bias to teacher expectancy effects. In: Dusek JB, Hall VC and Meyer WJ (eds) *Teacher Expectancies*. Erlbaum, Hillsdale, NJ.

2   McDermott I and Elfline J (2002) Personal communication. European NLP Coaching Certification Training. International Teaching Seminars, Essex.

3   Dilts R (1990) *Changing Belief Systems with Neurolinguistic Programming*. Meta Publications, Capitola, CA.

9

The secrets of success – the art of modelling

- How do we do what we actually do?
- How does one person excel where another remains just average?
- What is the difference that makes the difference?

This chapter will explore these questions and look at how we learn from each other. We will discover how to model successful strategies and how as coaches we can help the learner develop their strategies for improving or changing. We will build on what happens naturally by refining our skills of focusing, replacing judgement with curiosity and becoming specific and detailed.

Modelling is the term now used for the learning which occurs by watching another perform. We see it most commonly in children where they model behaviour and language from others around them. It takes place spontaneously and unconsciously without effort or deliberate intention to learn. On a recent skiing holiday to Canada one of our daughters, age nine, attended ski club (deliberately thus named rather than school). Within two days she was doing fast and neat parallel turns. When asked, she said all she'd done was play games, following fast behind and in the group leader's tracks. She was adamant that she had not been taught, she'd just done it because she could. Likewise, children in Guatemala learn to weave intricate patterns in exactly the same way – by sitting at their mothers' feet. This is modelling. Modelling is more than merely imitating. By getting inside behaviours and taking them on, the child makes them their own. In educational terms it relates directly to Albert Bandura's (1977) social learning theory. It refers to observational learning and is quite distinct from conditioning.[1]

As adults we continue to model, we model our peers or experts, even ourselves through videos. We model indirectly by asking ourselves questions such as, 'How would Dad have done this?' We have all had role models in certain areas who we aspire to. These are commonly teachers or co-professionals, but they may be icons such as the Dalai Lama or Winston Churchill. For others they are animals or inanimate objects who in metaphor represent skills that they desire. These may, for example, be mountains, trees, tigers or dolphins. Often our admiration for a role model, and our wish to emulate them remains just that, a wish, an idle musing which we do not actively pursue. So we dream on ... 'If only I could be like x, or if I could run to time like y then I would be OK.' Apprenticeships and master classes are an attempt to tap into this resource, to ask the questions, 'How does x do what he does?' and 'How will *you* be like x?' Coaching encourages and develops the skills of conscious modelling.

There is a shift now in education and business, such that modelling is becoming more and more recognised as being an extremely powerful tool. The skills of conscious modelling are being developed and increasingly taught. Modelling in business identifies key aspects that differentiate high performers, turning these aspects into an understandable and accessible framework, so helping others within the organisation adopt the same successful ways of working. The result is an improvement in achievement, satisfaction, effectiveness and financial output.

Modelling is generative; it assumes that every process has a *structure* which can be applied or adapted to any situation which is relevant. Making a cake, keeping to time, making someone welcome, running effective meetings, sleeping easy at night, relaxing, learning a new language, all have structures. These can be observed, sequenced and learnt. Similarly anxiety, pessimism and running late have structures. By exploring these structures, we can compare and contrast how we do things, so giving ourselves more choice in how we operate. We can tap into our own resources and avail ourselves of the expertise of others.

As a coach to your learner you are a powerful role model; your learner will unconsciously model your state, your curiosity and your ability to give feedback. They may ask you about specific skills and they will model how you cope with a variety of situations. If you know how to consciously model to improve your own performance, you can help them to refine what they do and what they choose to integrate into their behaviour.

Modelling what?

Modelling is the process of discovering the states, the way of thinking and the skills that enable someone to be a certain way or to accomplish a certain task. In order to model excellence we have to consider all the logical levels. It has been found that merely modelling and transferring behaviours does not bring long-term, sustainable change. Modelling is most successful when it is performed on all these different levels:

- environment
- behaviour
- capabilities
- beliefs and values
- sense of identity and purpose.

In modelling it is the last three levels where the 'the differences that make the difference' are usually found.

So, having realised this, we then have to choose what exactly it is we want to model. Here again the more specific and focused we can be about our desired outcome, the more likely we are to succeed. Our learning about outcome frames is invaluable here; we must have a clearly defined outcome, stated in the positive, with an evidence procedure for success.

For example a feasible modelling project may be, 'I want to model how he keeps calm and focused on the task in hand despite numerous interruptions.'

Imagine how much harder it would be to have a project to 'model how to be so generally laid back'. As a coach I would ask the learner to refine this by asking:

- What do you mean by being laid back?
- What do you actually see and hear him doing?
- Under what circumstances? With who? Who doesn't he do this with? When?
- How would you know if you were laid back? What would I actually see you doing? (evidence)
- So what is it you *actually* want to do?

Exercise

Think about a role model or someone you admire for their ability to do something a certain way or to be a particular way in a given situation.

1 Identify what it is specifically that you would like to do. How, where, when, with who?
2 Specify how it will serve you to do things in this way. This is very important – you can find out by asking yourself:

- How will this benefit me?
- Do I want this for myself?

- Do I believe that I can do this?
- Do I deserve this?

If the answer to any of the last three is no, then it is unlikely that you will succeed. Now is the time to rethink and refine what it is that you want.

3 Consider your evidence procedure. How will you know when you have succeeded? What will you be feeling, seeing, hearing doing? What will others notice?
4 Formulate a sentence to reflect what it is that you want: 'I want to model how to ...'

You will now have a well-formed outcome which is specific and concise and manageable. Indeed you may already have some ideas as to how this person does do what it is you are modelling.

How to model

The essentials

1 Establish and maintain rapport.
2 Be curious and interested ... suspend all judgement
3 Maintain a balance between conscious and unconscious, i.e. allow your mind to drift from time to time and just be.
4 Keep in mind your clear outcome and what your criteria for success are.
5 Maintain a set of filters to let you know what to pay attention to, and at what level of detail.

These really are essentials; if you just fire off loads of questions you will drown in a sea of meaningless information with no rudder to steer you to the still cove of integration and change.

The art

Lets us consider three aspects of the art of modelling:

1 *Ask*: 'What is the difference that makes the difference.' 'What are the key pieces? To do this, look for exceptions and counter examples, i.e. times when it doesn't work. In this way we determine the key elements of the behaviour, constructing a reproducible framework.

We must also get a behavioural demonstration, observing what happens. When we talk to someone and they are remembering what they do, you will learn some useful tips, but their memory and perception will almost certainly be different from their actual behavioural excellence. How many times have you seen this for yourself when you see yourself on video?

2   *Frame* modelling as an examination of behaviour (how do you do pre-exam nerves as opposed to pre-rugby match motivation?) rather than identity (why are you so anxious about exams when you're so focused in your rugby matches?). The structure of 'how we do things' is more amenable to change than the identity of 'who we are'. In this example, the question, 'Why are you so nervous about exams?' is likely to generate an answer such as 'I don't know' or 'I hate to put myself on the line'. Contrast this with the question, 'How do you do exam nerves?' which is likely to prompt answers such as, 'Well, I think about what it all means and I remember when I did really badly, then I feel sick and then I can't concentrate and I tell myself to pull myself together.' If we compare this to the more motivated state with rugby, it will be more useful: 'I enjoy it. I know it is not the end of the world whether we win or lose. I can see the faces of my team mates and let myself go.' We can now switch these positive states and behaviour to the negative situation of exam nerves. So, as a coach, the frame we use is one of ignorance and wonder, 'I'm really interested, how do you do that?' As the learner explains to us, they become clearer how they do things – their strategies for success and failure. We can then encourage them to compare and contrast these, so learning to use the positive strategies that they already have in a wider range of situations.

3   *Remember* that you are not trying to change yourself into someone else, you are you, *and* you are creating a new set of skills or way of being that you believe will have real benefit to you. It is like having a new wardrobe of clothes that you have tried on for size and you feel comfortable in, clothes that you can change in and out of depending on what you are doing. Modelling is really getting inside behaviour.

The specifics

Modelling requires the skills of focused observation and focused, specific questioning. Often the behaviours that we wish to model are performed by experts. Expert behaviour is unconscious or automatic – the person is often 'in flow', free of inhibition and self-judgement. When this happens, the mind does not act as a separate entity telling you what to do, or criticising, it is quiet and the expert feels 'together'. To ask someone who behaves in this way simply, 'How do you do that?' is likely to elicit the automatic response of 'I don't know', because they have lost their conscious knowing. Indeed, if they were to think and analyse, their behaviour may initially deteriorate. Think of tennis coaching where a new grip is suggested and you try to incorporate it into your automatic style ... as conscious thought steps in, more balls start to go out, and other aspects of your game are temporarily lost.

So in order to find out 'how' our observations must be acute and our questioning targeted.

The skill of observing

Conscious observation

We are often asked to observe others or ourselves, such as in a video recording, in order to feed back and learn. It is an acquired skill to able to observe and listen without judgement. It is easy to become so associated into events that we start thinking about what we would do or say, or we begin to anticipate reactions and inwardly cringe or celebrate. There are a few basic rules which, if adhered to, protect us from these natural human tendencies. These are:

- to remain physically detached or distanced from the situation
- to set the intention to just notice what happens and to suspend judgement
- to observe facts, to notice what happens, how things are said and what the sequence of events is without ascribing meaning
- to pay attention to detail
- to not assume anything.

In modelling we have to attune all our senses to register things that we may normally take for granted.

Unconscious observation – *'walking the walk'*

'Put yourself in his shoes' is a common saying, urging us to take another person's perspective. If we take this literally we can open ourselves to unconscious learning and observation. Try walking behind the person you are modelling, copying all that he or she does; take the same sized paces; move your head in the same way; notice where their arms and hands go; is there any sound; look where they look. This is a surprisingly powerful exercise. Immerse yourself completely, and notice how you are feeling. What is the self-talk in your head, what are you seeing and hearing? As we have already learnt, a person's physiological and mental state is a crucial factor in determining how they do things. This is a great way of getting into your model's state. For many people an aspect of this observed behaviour, be it posture or breathing or hand movements, becomes an anchor for them as they integrate the new behaviour into themselves.

The skill of focused questioning

Whenever we say or write things we always leave out detail – to include everything would take forever. So what we hear as interviewer is like the tip of an iceberg. In order to model successfully we must not assume what lies under the water, we need to clarify and expose further the nature of the iceberg. We need to listen carefully to what is vague in what the coachee is saying, to what is missing and to think about what beliefs or rules are underpinning their actions.

Consider these statements:

- I empty my head
- I think about it all day
- I get a clear understanding first
- I'm sure we all agree.

They are all missing content and meaning. You cannot assume meaning and content when modelling. Asking the right questions will help. What the right questions are depends on what you want to know and what you want to model. So we go back to our well-formed outcome.

Questions you may want to ask could include:

- You think about what, exactly?
- How do you think about it – do you have pictures, carry out self-talk, hear voices, feel something?
- What do you mean by all day? Every day?
- Are there times that you are not thinking about this?
- How does that affect you?
- Why is it important to do this?

We have looked in another chapter at meta-models (Chapter 7). The interventions we use to challenge deletions, distortions and generalisations are important in all modelling exercises. They are essential if we are to discover the specific detail of the 'how to'.

Example

Examples in modelling might include:

Deletion

I want to make a good impression	*How specifically do you want to impress?*
I feel passionate	*About what?*
It's much easier	*Than what? In which way is it easier?*

Generalisation

I never …	*Never?*
I have to reply to every call	*What would happen if you didn't?*
I can't show my feelings	*What stops you?*

Distortion

With that smile she must be popular	*How does her smiling make her popular?*
I know if they are annoyed	*What lets you know?*
The clock makes me tense	*How does it do that?*
It's fun to break rules	*Where does that come from?*

The structure of experience

Before we look at a framework of questions to use in modelling let us look at the structure of experience. Our senses are core to coding our experience, and we each have preferred senses that we use in different situations. The senses are interrelated – so, for example, a tone of voice may trigger a feeling felt somewhere in your body, a certain picture will be relaxing to one person and highly irritant to another, music creates moods. What are different are the links and the sequencing that we all use. Here is an example that the author found profound during neurolinguistic training with Ian McDermott, and which has changed her practice. It is an elegant example of modelling.

Example

During the Master Practitioner training, Ian read out an account by Rachel Remen of her experience of modelling by Carl Rogers:[2]

> Years ago, I was invited to a seminar given by Carl Rogers. I had never read his work but I knew that the seminar, attended by a group of therapists, was about 'unconditional positive regard'. At the time I was highly sceptical about this idea, but I attended the seminar anyway. I left transformed.
>
> Rogers' theories arose out of practice and his practice was intuitive and natural. In the seminar he tried to analyse what he was doing for us as he did it. He wanted to give a demonstration of unconditional positive regard in a therapeutic session. One of the therapists volunteered to serve as subject. As Rogers turned to the volunteer and was about to start the session, he suddenly pulled himself up, turned to us and said: 'I realise there's something I do before I start a session. I let myself know that I am enough. Not perfect. Perfect wouldn't be enough. There is nothing this man can do or say or feel that I can't feel in myself. I can be with him. I am enough'
>
> I was stunned by this. It felt as if some old wound in me, some fear of not being good enough, had come to an end. I knew, inside myself that what he said was absolutely true. I am not perfect, but I am enough.

This illustrates modelling at several levels. Carl Rogers is self-modelling, he tells the seminar how he structures his internal experience – *he lets himself know* that he is enough. He doesn't see himself working well, or feeling good, or imagining a scenario.

Remen was transformed by the experience and modelled herself on him; she let herself know that she is enough. Ian models the same thing throughout his training, and as a participant on his courses the effect was profound. It changed my clinical and coaching practice as I modelled it and it then became part of me. And there is another level too; if we as coaches behave as if we are human – not perfect, but enough – it follows that it is also enough for the learner to be human. What more enabling state can anyone ask for? So we can see how modelling becomes pivotal for effective learning, development and change.

Modelling around logical levels

Now we know the sort of experience and structure that we are looking to model, we can consider a framework of questions. This particular framework is based around the logical levels we discussed earlier. Again, depending on what it is you want to model, you may choose to concentrate on different areas. It is a pick list that is best used conversationally (I'm interested in ..., I wonder about ...). Slavishly working your way through the questions is not necessary. As you engage with your model you will find your own questions and search for detail that is important for you.

Exercise

Ask a friend or a family member to think about something they do well — maybe it is their hobby, or just something they do every day. Using your statement, 'I want to model how to do something or be a certain way that you do really well ...' Practise using some or all of these questions.

Environment
- What is important to you about your surroundings when you are doing this?
- What helps? What hinders?
- Where do you do this best? Where is it difficult?
- Is there anything that would stop you?

Behaviour
- What do you actually do? (It is important here to look for sequencing.)
- What do you do first? Then what do you do?
- What do you do beforehand? How do you prepare?
- What do you do afterwards? How do you know when you are done? How do you let go?
- When do you do this? Is there a time that you don't do this?

Capabilities
- How do you do this?
- What are you thinking?
- What are you saying to yourself?
- What do you see? What do you hear?
- What do you feel?
- What resources do you have which help you?

- What helps you? What hinders you?
- And of all of these, which is the one that you couldn't do without or without which this wouldn't work?
- What would it take to make you even better at this?

Beliefs and values
- What is important about this for you?
- What do you believe about this?
- What values are you honouring by doing this?

Sense of identity and purpose
- Who are you being when you do this?
- What does it say about you?
- What is your intention when you do this?
- Why do you do this?
- What is your purpose in doing this?

The uses and value of modelling

We learn from story telling, from doing and from copying. We have being learning like this unconsciously since we were children. In modelling as adults, we develop a framework whereby we can continue to grow and develop more systematically. We expand our options of how to behave in different situations and can try different ways on for size until we find the 'coat' that fits us best. As a coach and teacher, it is an invaluable way of learning new skills for ourselves. It also offers opportunities for our learners. Imagine now how you will respond when a learner asks you, 'How did you do that?' Using the framework you have just learnt you can guide them through the different aspects, or you can suggest things that they might like to look for that even you are unaware of. And so they will start modelling, looking and asking as the child did when they began to ski – without having had to go to school and 'learn'.

Another use of modelling is to analyse and adapt existing strategies for ourselves or for our learners. Modelling our own successes and transferring the skills to new areas makes sense: we are our own best teacher and we have a stack of personal resources ... it's just that we don't always tap into this. Reflective learning is a step in this direction, but it often falls short by stopping at the stage of analysis. In many people's minds, an understanding of why something happens, with a greater awareness of the issues involved leads automatically to behaviour change. They then seem surprised when it happens all over again. We are all familiar with the refrain, 'I know why I do it and I know I shouldn't, but I just can't help it.' Milton Erickson is reputed to have said, 'Change leads to insight far more often than insight leads to change'. Modelling gets away from the *why* into the *how*. Let us look at how we can model our own success.

'Me as my model': the secrets of my success

If we presuppose that behaviour is a set of learnt skills and beliefs, then we can see ourselves as capable, as having the right set of skills to behave in that way. Now it may be that our current skills are not being used in the most appropriate way or circumstances. A modelling mindset enables us to be curious, non-judgemental and to take a dispassionate view of what is going on. So we are able to compare and contrast what works and what doesn't.

How often have you examined what it is you do well and transferred the skills over to a new area? Has your partner ever commented on how you can be so organised or empathetic at work, and then you come home and behave in the opposite way? Wouldn't it be great to break down the structure of this behaviour and use it in other areas of your life? There are many similar examples. The consultant who easily makes conversation at business lunches and yet sits alone at drinks parties given by neighbours; the efficient personal assistant whose wardrobe and handbag is bulging in disorganisation; the assertive professional who gets upset and avoids conflict outside work; the musician who loves playing in a band but goes to pieces at interviews. The more we look, the more we see how we can be our own teacher, our model. To do this we must become curious about the structure of our own experience, and we need to give ourselves the positive unconditional regard that Carl Rogers used with his clients. Entrepreneurs are naturally good at this, yet for many other people it can seem like a tall order. As a coach you have the opportunity to demonstrate positive unconditional regard to your learner and to show them how to model themselves. This will be the most important tool for professional and personal development that you can give anyone.

As a coach you enable your learner to see that behaviour is a learnt response which relates in specific and appropriate ways to life experience. Behaviour becomes controllable and changeable without damaging the integrity of self. The learner will often bring to his coach an experience of behaviour that did not work well. You will be able to examine this with them and also to compare and contrast it to behaviour that does work. Once the structure of successful experience is known, the learner's own success structures can be replicated and transferred to other contexts. Once learnt, this process of self-modelling, of looking for effectiveness, can be carried out by the learners themselves.

Example

Let us consider an example from a coaching scenario, where the coachee (an experienced professional) was feeling very nervous about a forthcoming assessment visit as she had failed the viva part of her last exam first time round. She felt that she should pull herself together and prepare 'properly' for the visit.

Coach: Can you tell me how it is when you think about preparing for this visit. What happens exactly?

Coachee: Well, its horrible, when I start to think about it I feel sick and sweaty, then I tell myself to pull myself together and just get on with it, it will be fine … except I don't believe it will be fine.

Coach: So you are feeling sick. Tell me more about that, where is it, what is it like?

Coachee: Well, here, in the pit of my stomach, I feel paralysed. My mind goes blank.

Coach: And feeling paralysed and blank you tell yourself …

Coachee: Yes, in this really cross voice and then I get even crosser for wasting time and energy.

Coach: So even thinking about preparing for this visit sounds like very hard work, not a motivating experience. So then what happens?

Coachee: I get up, make some tea, tidy the desk, look at the clock and decide I'll do it tomorrow.

Coach: OK so you put it all off.

Coachee: Yes …

Coach: I'm interested – can you tell me about a time when you enjoyed preparing for something?

Coachee (after a long pause): Yes, I really enjoy preparing for the local pantomime, it's scary being on stage but I love the buzz, I can see me up there with all my makeup on, I can hear the audience laughing and singing and I just know I'll feel tired but fantastic.

Coach: You imagine how it is going to be, you see it like a film?

Coachee: Yes, sort of, except I'm in it – I feel worthwhile, part of something bigger. If I'm tired after work and am not sure about rehearsal, I just imagine how it will be.

Coach: So preparing for something you enjoy doing, you first imagine, see a picture, then you feel the buzz and you hear the audience?

Coachee: Yes – I feel energised.

Coach: So that's a strategy that works for you.

Coachee: Yes.

Coach: And is there anything else?

Coachee: Yes … I know I'm OK − I can do this.

Coach: Ah, great − so you have something that works and we know that it's different from the strategy that doesn't work … with that one you don't believe you can do it and you feel sick. With this one you see yourself succeeding and having fun from the sounds of things. You hear others' positive reactions and you feel energised knowing you can do it. So what has to happen now for you to prepare for this assessment visit, to see yourself performing well, hearing a positive response knowing that you can do it …? See how good that is … notice how it is to believe that you can do this …

The session continues by structuring a new experience of preparation by creating an image and a state of 'can do'. The coachee subsequently reported being creative in her preparation and actually enjoying and learning something from her assessment visit.

In a coaching relationship there are many opportunities to compare and contrast experience in this way. So the learner gains confidence, they remain congruent as they develop new approaches and also become more open and curious to learn about how other people do it. There is a kindness and tolerance that comes with modelling, as we discover that we are all expert, and all human. We can start to do this for ourselves.

Exercise

Self-modelling − comparing and contrasting

To do this exercise make sure you are somewhere relaxed and comfortable, give yourself time and put yourself in a state of mind of just wondering, idly mulling over, not looking for right or wrong. Give yourself permission to smile and laugh with yourself.

Pick one from the following and compare and contrast for yourself the sequence and nature of experience by focusing on how you feel, what you are saying to yourself, what you see, what you hear and what you believe. Think of real examples and examine the detail of how it happens for you.

- A time when you were confused, compared to a time when you were certain.
- A time where a difficulty appeared to be a problem, compared to when you treated a difficulty as an opportunity.

- A circumstance where you felt indifferent, compared to one where you were motivated.
- An event where you considered yourself a failure, compared to an event where you saw yourself as a success.

Notice how you feel. What do you see and hear? What do you tell yourself? What do others see? What comes first, and then what? You may cycle round in circles, or it may be a straight jump from one to another. Find the 'difference that is the difference' for you between the two events. It may help you to keep notes.

Now think about the situation that could have been different, such as being confused. In your mind's eye, transfer the sequence and structure of the successful way of doing it to the less successful way. So, for example, run the time when you were confused, using the sequences and structures of the times when you were certain. Create and practise your new experience in your mind's eye. Run a video with sound track so you see and hear yourself using the successful strategy. This is you ...

Conclusion

Modelling is the most natural way of learning and developing. It is also one of the oldest methods of teaching; it is what Socrates did by asking questions, it is what apprentices do when working alongside an expert. The difference here is that we have transferred modelling from unconscious to conscious awareness, acknowledging it as a powerful process. By applying modelling to ourselves and our learners, we offer more choice with a greater flexibility of behaviour, more tolerance and more curiosity in our humanness.

References

1   Bandura A (1977) *Social Learning Theory*. Prentice-Hall, Englewood Cliffs, NJ.

2   Remen R (1989) The search for healing. In: Carlson R and Shield B (eds) *Healers on Healing*. Jeremy P Tarcher, Los Angeles, CA, p. 930.

10

And finally

The framework of coaching is very honouring to the individual learner, and to the process of continuing personal and professional development. The coaching approach to learning is Socratic; it uses questions that come from a position of curiosity and non-judgment, to enable learners to learn for themselves.

The concepts and techniques you have read about may sound easy and obvious. In many ways they are, and, in many ways they are not. As teachers, we too are constantly learning and developing. We have our own beliefs and values which may limit us. The phrase 'easier said than done' springs to mind as being highly relevant to actually using coaching skills. We would urge you not to just say 'oh yes that's all obvious' and leave the book to gather dust and be a tick in your own learning portfolio. We would urge you to really practise the techniques, to notice what aspects of teaching challenge you, and to use the book as a resource that you dip in and out of. And as you do this be kind to yourself, set yourself one new skill to practise at a time, write it in your diary and give yourself at least a week with each, so that you really start to become fluent and flexible in applying coaching to teaching. And as you do this, allow yourself to have fun and to be curious.

We believe that coaching skills can complement and augment traditional teaching methods. They are not to be used instead of, but as well as. There are times when a learner is very self-directed and motivated in gaining information and skills and passing exams; here the emphasis is on coaching to encourage ongoing personal and professional development at a much deeper level. However, there are also times when a coaching approach is not appropriate; there may be issues of basic professional incompetence that must be addressed, or the learner may not be ready or willing to engage, or you may not have the energy to work at this level at a particular time in your life or with a particular individual. You as teacher are free to choose when and with whom you use these skills.

The coaching skills you will develop in teaching are also transferable to other parts of your life. They are useful in such diverse areas as running and contributing in meetings, negotiating with colleagues and family, dealing with teenagers, managing teams. The coaching perspective is valuable in all areas of life. We hope that you have enjoyed this book and that you will take from it something of meaning and of value to you.

Index

Page numbers in italics refer to figures or tables.